C000172272

VEGE

COOKBOOK FOR

BEGINNERS 2023

The Ultimate Guide to a

Successful and Fresh Vegetarian

Diet

EMILY HARTMAN

TABLE OF CONTENTS

Introduction

Greetings and welcome to the exciting world of plant-based culinary delights! In today's ever-evolving landscape of dietary preferences and choices, adopting a vegetarian lifestyle has gained immense popularity and traction due to its myriad of remarkable benefits. Whether you have decided to embrace vegetarianism for health motivations, environmental concerns, ethical considerations, or simply to explore thrilling new flavors and dishes, the Vegetarian Cookbook for Beginners 2023 is your comprehensive guide to embarking on a flavorful, nutritious and rewarding plant-based journey.

This cookbook is specifically designed and tailored for individuals who are new to the vegetarian lifestyle and are eager to discover the magnificent art of plant-based cooking. It provides a wealth and plethora of mouth-watering, simple to follow vegetarian recipes that will inspire, energize and delight your taste buds while also promoting a healthier, more sustainable and eco-friendly lifestyle. With a primary focus on simplicity, accessibility, inclusivity and optimal nutrition, this book aims to properly equip you with the requisite knowledge, skills, tips and techniques to create vibrant, colorful, satisfying meatless meals in the comfort of your own kitchen.

Let this cookbook be your trusted companion as you explore the versatile, vibrant world of vegetarian cuisine! An exciting culinary adventure awaits you.

The Vegetarian Cookbook for Beginners 2023 is thoughtfully crafted and designed to specifically cater to the unique needs and challenges faced by individuals who are in the process of transitioning to and adopting a vegetarian diet. Whether you are a complete culinary novice who has rarely stepped foot in the kitchen, or a seasoned cook with ample experience looking to expand your horizons into the vibrant plant-based cuisine world, this book offers a comprehensive, thorough introduction covering the fundamental principles, techniques, ingredients, and skills required to excel at vegetarian cooking.

Within the pages of this guide, you will find a diverse array of insights and information to properly equip you on your vegetarian cooking journey, regardless of your current skill level. Core vegetarian cooking concepts such as balancing flavors, textures, colors and nutrients in the absence of meat are explained in a simple, understandable manner. You will learn about the array of wholesome plant-based ingredients that serve as the foundation of vegetarian cuisine, from various types of vegetables, grains and legumes to eggs and dairy if you pursue a lacto-ovo vegetarian diet. Additionally, the book provides guides on essential techniques such as roasting, sautéing, baking, pressure cooking, marinating and more using plant-based ingredients.

Whether you are seeking to improve your overall health, reduce your environmental footprint, or simply discover new culinary horizons, the Vegetarian Cookbook for Beginners 2023 serves as the perfect guide to transition you into the satisfying, flavorful world of vegetarian cooking. Let this book open your eyes to an exciting plant-based journey!

Key Features:

Embark on a fulfilling culinary and nutritional journey into vegetarianism with this comprehensive cookbook tailored to guide and empower beginners.

The cookbook begins with an in-depth, practical introduction to the principles, varied types, and remarkable benefits of plant-based eating so you can start your vegetarian transition with a solid, clear understanding. Explore the spectrum of vegetarian diets, from lacto-ovo to vegan. Learn about essential vitamins, minerals and nutrients to watch for, along with useful meal planning strategies, grocery shopping tips, and lifestyle advice to ensure a balanced, enjoyable and sustainable shift.

At the heart of the cookbook lies lots of mouthwatering, innovative recipes thoughtfully crafted to appeal to diverse tastes and preferences. From vibrant, nourishing breakfasts and protein-packed mains to decadent desserts and refreshing beverages, each recipe delights and showcases the astounding versatility of vegetarian ingredients. The recipes cater to beginner cooks through clear, step-by-step instructions and helpful tips, but also contain enough flair to entice more seasoned chefs.

The cookbook further equips you with indispensable vegetarian cooking knowledge, from essential equipment, to ingredient selection, storage and preparation, to core cooking techniques tailored specifically to plant-based ingredients. Learn how to coax the maximum flavor and nutrition out of each vegetable, grain and legume while also discovering substitutes for common animal products.

This thoughtful vegetarian guide truly empowers beginners to feel confident and creative in the kitchen. Immerse yourself in an enriching culinary journey as you develop skills, explore new produce and flavors, adapt recipes to your tastes, and embrace the joys of plant-based eating. Let this cookbook open your eyes to the colorful, flavorful world of vegetarian cuisine!

Chapter One

The Basics of Vegetarian

Cooking

Vegetarianism is the practice of abstaining from the consumption of meat, and may also include abstention from by-products of animal slaughter. Vegetarianism can be adopted for various reasons including health, ethics, environmentalism, culture, aesthetics or taste. There are several forms of vegetarianism:

Lacto vegetarianism involves abstaining from meat, fish, and eggs, but allows the consumption of dairy products. This form of

13

vegetarianism is based on ethical reasons of avoiding harm to animals, as well as health reasons, since dairy products are a good source of calcium and protein. However, the production of milk still involves some cruelty and exploitation of cows.

Ovo vegetarianism involves abstaining from all meat and dairy, but allows the consumption of eggs. Like lacto vegetarianism, this diet contains a good source of protein from eggs, but avoids the ethical issues associated with dairy farming. However, egg production still causes harm to chickens.

Lacto-ovo vegetarianism (or ovo-lacto vegetarianism) involves abstaining from meat, fish and seafood, but allows the consumption of dairy products and eggs. This is one of the most common forms of vegetarianism. By avoiding meat but allowing eggs and dairy, it provides a balanced diet containing complete proteins. However, ethical issues with the dairy and egg industries remain.

Pescatarianism involves abstaining from the consumption of meat and poultry, but allows fish and seafood. Eggs and dairy may also be consumed. This diet is based on health reasons, as fish is a good source of omega-3 fatty acids, as well as ethical reasons, as fishing may be considered less unethical than farming practices of land animals. However, there are still ethical issues with commercial fishing.

Pollotarianism involves abstaining from consuming meat from mammals and fish, but allows poultry and other fowl. Eggs and dairy may also be consumed. The rationale is that chickens and other birds are less cognitively complex than mammals. However, poultry farming remains quite inhumane in industrial systems.

Flexitarianism involves abstaining from meat for the most part, but occasionally includes meat in one's diet. This allows for greater flexibility and accessibility than strict vegetarianism, but still reduces the overall consumption of meat for environmental and ethical reasons. However, it does not completely eliminate the issues associated with meat production.

Veganism is one of the strictest forms of vegetarianism, abstaining from the consumption or use of any products derived from animals, including meat, seafood, poultry, eggs, dairy, honey, leather, wool, silk, etc. Veganism is practiced for strong ethical reasons, opposing animal cruelty and exploitation. However, it requires meticulous checking of ingredients to avoid animal by-products.

Raw veganism involves consuming only plant foods that are uncooked, unprocessed, and often organic or wild-sourced. The rationale is that cooking foods depletes nutrients and enzymes. However, nutritional balance may be difficult to achieve, and some foods contain compounds that are toxic or difficult to digest when raw.

Fruitarianism is an extreme form of raw veganism that restricts the diet to primarily fruits, nuts and seeds. Avoiding vegetables, grains and protein-rich plant foods can make it challenging to meet nutritional needs. Long-term fruitarianism carries health risks like malnutrition.

As we can see, vegetarianism has several variations, stemming from different motivations like ethics, environment, health, culture or taste preferences. Complete avoidance of animal products requires the most strict adherence, while allowing eggs, dairy or certain meats provides more flexibility and nutritional balance. However, even partial vegetarianism can reduce the environmental impact and ethical issues associated with intensive animal farming. The most suitable form depends on each individual's ethical values and nutritional needs.

Benefits of a vegetarian diet for health, the environment, and animal welfare.

A vegetarian diet, which avoids meat and fish, can have significant benefits for health, the environment, and animal welfare. Below we highlight some of the main advantages.

Health Benefits:

Studies show that well-planned vegetarian diets are healthy for all stages of life. They tend to be lower in saturated fat and cholesterol, and higher in fruits, vegetables, whole grains, legumes, nuts and soy products. This results in reduced risk of chronic diseases like heart disease, type 2 diabetes, obesity, and certain cancers.

Vegetarians typically have lower BMI and obesity levels, lower blood pressure and cholesterol, and reduced rates of hypertension and type 2 diabetes. Plant-based diets are linked to higher intakes of beneficial nutrients like fiber, antioxidants, magnesium, potassium, folate and vitamin C.

Additionally, vegetarians exhibit lower rates of cataracts, diverticulitis, gallstones, kidney stones, osteoporosis, rheumatoid arthritis and dementia. If well-planned, vegetarian diets can meet all nutritional needs and support healthy growth and development in children.

Environmental Benefits:

Adopting vegetarian diets combats climate change and environmental degradation. Animal agriculture generates more greenhouse gas emissions than transport. It also requires massive amounts of land, water and energy compared to plant foods.

If the global population shifted to a vegetarian diet, food-related emissions could be cut by 63%, and total emissions cut by 29%. Land use for agriculture could be reduced by 75%, freeing up land for ecosystems and wildlife. Water usage could be cut by 19%, helping conserve this precious resource.

The biodiversity impacts would also be significant - expansion of pasture and croplands for animal feed is a leading cause of deforestation and species extinction. Shifting away from meat allows more sustainable plant-based agriculture.

Animal Welfare Benefits:

Perhaps the most direct impact of vegetarianism is on the billions of animals farmed and killed for food each year. Animal welfare is severely compromised in industrial farming systems to maximize productivity and profits. Chickens, cows, pigs and fish often suffer extreme confinement, deprivation, mutilations and stress.

By avoiding meat and animal products, vegetarians withdraw support for these cruel systems. Widespread vegetarianism would decrease demand for meat and encourage farms to shift to more humane practices. While some animal suffering would still exist, the scale of animal cruelty and slaughter would be greatly diminished through diet change.

The evidence shows vegetarian diets can support human health, environmental sustainability, and improved animal welfare. Avoiding our overreliance on meat has interlinked benefits across these domains. While viable for people at all life stages, vegetarianism does require planning to ensure nutritional needs are met, especially for children. Overall, reducing society's demand for animal products would lead to significant positive impacts.

Meal planning tips

Planning nutritious and satisfying vegetarian meals requires some knowledge and effort, especially for beginners. Here are some tips to make vegetarian meal planning and grocery shopping easier:

- Build meals around vegetables, fruits, whole grains, legumes, nuts and plant-based proteins like tofu. This ensures you get fiber, antioxidants, healthy fats and key nutrients.

- Include a protein source like legumes, tofu, tempeh, edamame or nuts/seeds with each meal. Combining plants provides complete proteins.

- Don't forget healthy fats from oils, nuts, seeds and avocados for energy and nutrient absorption.

- Read labels and choose whole, unprocessed options instead of refined, sugary foods. Limit highly processed meat and dairy substitutes.

- Plan for variety and rotate different plant-based protein sources throughout the week like beans, lentils, chickpeas, tofu etc.

- Make large batches of whole grains like brown rice or quinoa to use throughout the week for easy meals.

- Get creative with tofu, seitan, tempeh - marinate and roast, crumble, stir fry or blend into dishes for different flavors.

- Use egg replacements like flax eggs or bananas to bake vegetarian treats and goods.

- Stock up on versatile frozen, canned and dried vegetables, fruits, beans and lentils to pull together quick meals.

- Plan make-ahead breakfasts and lunches like overnight oats, tofu scrambles, roasted veggie and hummus wraps.

Grocery Shopping Tips

- Stick to the perimeter for fresh produce, dairy/dairy alternatives, bulk bins of grains and nuts.

- Stock up on versatile ingredients: beans, lentils, nuts, seeds, whole grains, spices, herbs, plant-based milks and yogurts.

27

- Seek out whole food sources of plant protein: tofu, tempeh, edamame, seitan, beans, lentils, chickpeas.

- Check labels for hidden animal ingredients like gelatin, casein, albumin, whey if following strict vegetarian/vegan diets.

- Buy multi-purpose ingredients to use in different recipes throughout the week.

- Purchase nutrient-dense superfoods like quinoa, hemp seeds, chia seeds, nutritional yeast.

- Limit processed meat substitutes and cheeses which are often high in sodium and additives.

- Buy organic produce if your budget allows to reduce pesticide exposure. Prioritize the "Dirty Dozen".

- Get colorful produce to maximize phytonutrient and antioxidant intake.

Building a Balanced Vegetarian Diet

- Include a daily protein source: beans, lentils, tofu, tempeh, edamame, nuts, seeds, quinoa etc.

- Eat a rainbow of fruits and vegetables for fiber, vitamins, minerals. Aim for 7-9 servings per day.

- Incorporate whole grains and limit refined carbs: oats, brown rice, barley, bran cereal, whole grain bread.

29

- Don't avoid fats. Include healthy unsaturated fats from olive oil, avocados, nuts and seeds.

- Choose fortified plant-based milks, yogurts and cereals to obtain calcium, vitamin D and B12.

- Consider a Vitamin B12 supplement if not consuming dairy or fortified foods. Also vit D if sunshine exposure is low.

- Stay hydrated with water and herbal teas. Limit sugary drinks.

With proper meal planning strategies, grocery shopping know-how and balanced diet principles, vegetarians can meet all their nutritional needs. It may take some extra work initially, but a plant-based diet can easily become habit with the right techniques and staple ingredients readily on hand. With a little education, vegetarian diets are nutritious and sustainable lifelong.

Cooking Techniques

Cooking vegetarian dishes requires knowing how to best bring out flavors and textures in fruits, vegetables, grains, legumes and other plant-based ingredients. Here is an overview of cooking techniques frequently used in vegetarian cuisine:

Sautéing

Sautéing involves quickly cooking foods in a minimal amount of fat, like oil or butter, over relatively high heat. The food is kept moving constantly. Sautéing brings out flavors and nicely browns or caramelizes foods. It works well for denser vegetables like broccoli, carrots, peppers and zucchini. Just take care not to overcook more delicate veggies. Sautéing is also good for tofu, tempeh and seitan.

Stir-Frying

Stir-frying is similar to sautéing but at even higher heat and with faster cooking in a wok or skillet. Chopped ingredients are added in succession starting with those needing the longest cooking time. Stir-frying preserves crunch and bright flavors in veggies. A flavorful sauce is often added just at the end. It's important to have all ingredients prepped before stir-frying to keep the cooking fast-paced.

Roasting

Roasting involves cooking vegetables, fruits, beans or meat alternatives like tofu uncovered in the oven, allowing surfaces to caramelize. Natural sugars concentrate creating deeper, sweeter flavors. A light coating of oil helps facilitate browning. Heartier vegetables like potatoes, carrots, parsnips and cauliflower especially shine with high oven heat. Roasting brings out natural sweetness.

Steaming

Steaming involves suspending foods like vegetables or dumplings in a basket over boiling water. The heat of the steam cooks the food. This moist-heat method preserves nutrients better than boiling and keeps colors and flavors vibrant. Steaming is suited for more delicate produce like broccoli, green beans, kale and snap peas.

Braising

Braising involves browning ingredients then slowly simmering them in a small amount of liquid like broth, wine or sauce. The gentle moist heat tenderizes vegetables, fruits, beans or denser proteins like seitan, tempeh or tofu. Braising enhances flavor as seasonings meld together with the cooking liquid reducing into a sauce. Slow cooking times vary from 30 minutes to a few hours depending on the ingredients.

Grilling

Grilling imparts a delicious charred flavor. Vegetables, fruits, marinated tofu, tempeh or portobello mushrooms can be grilled over a hot open flame or heated grill. Grilling brings out sweetness in vegetables and fruits through caramelization. Natural sugars in marinades also caramelize adding flavor. Grilling adds appetizing smoky flavors from the licking flames.

Baking

Baking uses prolonged dry heat in an oven to cook vegetables, casseroles, grains or baked goods like breads, cakes and cookies. Baking brings out natural sweetness and deeply concentrates flavors in veggies. The dry heat of baking creates a nice crust on items like tofu or casseroles. Vegetarian baking utilizes egg substitutes, plant-based milks and oils in place of dairy products.

Air Frying

Air frying uses extremely hot, circulating air to produce a crispy, browned exterior similar to deep frying. With little or no oil needed, it is a healthier cooking method. Air frying gives vegetarian foods like tofu, tempeh, falafel and vegetables a satisfying crunch. It also nicely crisps sides like fritters and fried vegetables. Air frying requires frequent shaking or tossing for even cooking.

Vegetarian cooking uses a range of techniques like sautéing, roasting, braising, grilling and baking to transform fruits, vegetables and other plant foods into delicious dishes. Knowing when to apply the proper cooking method brings out the best flavors, textures and aromas.

Use of herbs and spices

Herbs and spices are invaluable for adding flavor, aroma and depth to vegetarian dishes. Mastering their use can elevate simple ingredients into boldly seasoned plant-based meals. Below are tips on incorporating herbs and spices for maximum impact:

Fresh Herbs

Fresh herbs like basil, cilantro, parsley, mint, dill and oregano supply brightness and herbaceous notes. Add them at the end of cooking or as garnish so their flavor isn't diminished. Chopped fresh herbs complement grains, beans, soups, salads, sauces, dressings and dips. Large leafy herbs can be torn or left whole for visual appeal. Delicate soft herbs like basil, mint and cilantro should be added just before serving. Heartier herbs like thyme, rosemary and oregano can be added earlier in cooking.

Dried Herbs

Dried herbs have concentrated flavor so use smaller amounts compared to fresh. Add them early when simmering soups, stews and sauces so the flavors infuse. Italian seasoning contains basil, oregano and rosemary,while herbs de Provence includes lavender, fennel and marjoram. Use dried thyme, oregano, dill and parsley in bean dishes, lentils and vegetarian roasts. Avoid dried herbs in uncooked preparations as their texture diminishes freshness.

Spice Blends

Premade spice blends eliminate measuring many separate spices. Blends like garam masala, Chinese five spice, ras el hanout and za'atar include warming spices like cumin, cardamom, cinnamon and coriander. Use them to season lentils, beans, veggies, tofu or tempeh. Curry powder can add exotic flair and turmeric's golden color and mild flavor complements many dishes. Pump up chili powder, cumin and paprika in Tex-Mex recipes.

Warmed Spices

Blooming spices briefly in hot oil or butter releases their essential oils and intensifies their flavors. Warming cumin, coriander and mustard seeds adds nutty depth to Indian curries and dals. Blooming cinnamon and cardamom enhances their sweetness in oatmeal, curries and baked goods. Sauté ginger and garlic before adding wet ingredients for heightened aroma.

Spice Rubs and Marinades

Combine spices with oil, vinegar and fresh herbs to make zesty marinades for tofu, tempeh, mushrooms or eggplant. Chili powder, cumin, paprika and oregano add boldness to Mexican marinades. Or blend curry powder, coriander, cumin and ginger for an Indian flare. Grill or roast the food after marinating to caramelize the spices and marry the flavors.

Spice Pastes

Make a wet spice paste to amp up the flavor of sautéed or stir-fried dishes. In a blender or mortar and pestle, finely grind garlic, fresh chilies, ginger and lemongrass with splash of water or oil to form a paste. Spice pastes provide a flavor base for Thai and Indian vegetarian fare before adding vegetables, grains or beans.

Seeds and Pepper

Poppy, caraway, sesame and fennel seeds provide nutty flavors and crunch when sprinkled on salads, rice, baked goods or roasted veggies. Crushed peppercorns add biting heat while whole peppercorns lend mild floral spice. Allspice berries complement sweet baking while star anise enhances Asian noodle broths.

Herbs and spices allow you to add punch, depth, complexity and character to plant-based meals. A world of flavors awaits your experiments with different seasoning combos. Start with small amounts, taste and adjust. Varying herbs and spices ensures vegetarian food is anything but bland.

Chapter Two

Nutritional Info

In the past few years, there has been a noticeable uptick in the number of people adopting a vegetarian diet. This meat-free way of eating has attracted many devotees due to its promotion of health, compassion for animals, and sustainability. At its core, a vegetarian diet is characterized by plant-based foods like fruits, vegetables, beans, lentils, whole grains, nuts and seeds. Meat, poultry, fish and seafood are excluded. The purpose of this chapter is to take an in-depth look at the immense nutritional benefits possible on a well-balanced vegetarian diet. It will highlight the plethora of essential vitamins, minerals, and other nutrients available from vegetarian food sources. Additionally, common misconceptions about the ability of plant-based diets to meet human nutritional requirements will be debunked.

To start, it is important to define what constitutes a vegetarian diet. There are several levels of vegetarianism. Lacto-ovo vegetarians consume dairy products and eggs but no meat, poultry or seafood. A vegan diet eliminates all animal products including dairy, eggs, honey and gelatin. Vegetarians who include fish in their diet are known as pescatarians. And many self-described vegetarians occasionally eat meat, chicken or fish, meaning they follow a flexitarian or semi-vegetarian diet. No matter the type, vegetarian diets emphasize nutrient-dense whole plant foods.

When well-planned, vegetarian diets are considered appropriate for all stages of life, including pregnancy, lactation, infancy, childhood, adolescence and old age. Research shows that vegetarian diets can provide significant benefits for health. Vegetarians generally have lower body mass index, lower cholesterol levels, lower blood pressure levels and less incidence of heart disease, type 2 diabetes and certain types of cancer. The fiber-rich nature of plant foods promotes digestive and cardiovascular health. And the abundance of beneficial plant compounds, like antioxidants and phytochemicals, contribute to longevity and wellbeing.

Some people mistakenly assume that important nutrients like protein, iron, calcium, vitamin D, vitamin B12 and omega-3 fatty acids are lacking or insufficient in vegetarian diets. However, there are plentiful plant-based sources for all of these. For protein, options include legumes, nuts, seeds, whole grains, dairy products, eggs (for lacto-ovo vegetarians) and soy foods like tofu. Iron is found in beans, lentils, spinach and fortified grains and cereals. Calcium-rich foods include dark green leafy vegetables, almonds, figs, fortified plant milks

47

and yogurts. Vitamin D comes from sunlight, fortified milks and mushrooms. Vitamin B12 is obtained via fortified foods, nutritional yeast and supplements. And alpha-linolenic acid, an omega-3 fat, exists in plant oils, nuts, seeds and soy. With mindful meal planning, vegetarians can easily fulfill all their nutritional requirements.

Some key considerations when following a vegetarian diet include consuming sufficient calories, eating a rainbow of fruits and vegetables, choosing whole nutritious sources of protein, incorporating adequate fats and oils, and supplementing when necessary with items like vitamin B12. Variety is paramount so that nutrient needs are met across the food groups.

A day's meals may include oatmeal with fruit for breakfast, a black bean and veggie burrito for lunch, lentil soup and whole grain bread for dinner, and mixed nuts for a snack. With endless possible combinations incorporating colorful produce, whole grains, beans, nuts and seeds, the vegetarian diet provides limitless options for creating nutrient-rich and satisfying meals.

Scientific evidence consistently shows that balanced vegetarian diets have extensive health advantages, decreasing risk for many chronic diseases and conditions. When meticulously planned, vegetarians can consume all the necessary vitamins, minerals and macronutrients needed for optimal functioning. In fact, some studies suggest vegetarians often surpass non-vegetarians in overall intake of protective nutrients like antioxidants and phytochemicals that promote longevity. While requiring attention to ensure adequate nutrition, the vegetarian diet is a highly nutritious and health-promoting way of eating that is suitable for people in all phases of life. With its many benefits for health, ethics and the environment, it is likely that adoption of meat-free eating plans will only continue to expand in upcoming years.

Carbohydrates are a macronutrient that serves as the primary fuel source for the body. They exist in abundance within a well-planned vegetarian diet. Carbohydrates are found in whole grains like brown rice, quinoa, oats, barley and whole wheat bread and pasta. Starchy vegetables including potatoes, sweet potatoes, corn and winter squash also provide carbohydrates. Fruits of all kinds are carbohydrate sources, with options like bananas, apples, oranges, grapes and melons. Legumes, including beans, lentils, chickpeas and peas are another vegetarian carb choice. These complex carbohydrates break down into glucose during digestion, which the body then uses for energy production and fueling the brain and muscles.

Beyond energy, the carbohydrates in the vegetarian diet confer additional benefits. Fiber is a type of carbohydrate that promotes digestive and cardiovascular health by aiding elimination, maintaining bowel regularity, reducing blood cholesterol and controlling blood sugar. Whole grains, fruits, vegetables and legumes all contain high levels of beneficial fiber. Carbohydrates also assist with weight management and appetite control when consumed in appropriate portions. And diets rich in plant-based carbohydrates have been associated with reduced risks for chronic diseases like type 2 diabetes, heart disease and certain cancers. For optimal health, vegetarians should base their meals around minimally processed, whole food sources of carbohydrates.

Protein is another essential macronutrient needed by the body for growth, tissue repair, enzyme production and more. Traditionally, animal products like meat, eggs and dairy were considered the ideal protein sources due to their complete amino acid profiles. However, by eating a varied diet, vegetarians can also easily meet all of their protein needs from plant-based sources alone. Legumes including beans, lentils, chickpeas, peas and peanuts are great choices, providing around 15 grams protein per cooked cup. Tofu, tempeh and seitan supply about 20 grams per a serving. Ancient grains like quinoa and amaranth contain approximately 8 grams protein per cooked cup, as do nuts and nut butters. Hemp seeds, chia seeds, spinach, asparagus, artichokes, broccoli and potatoes are other vegetarian protein sources.

Through combinations like rice and beans, whole grain pasta with lentils, oatmeal with nuts or veggie burgers on whole wheat buns, plant proteins can complement each other to provide all the essential amino acids required by the body. Studies show that plant-based diets can adequately support protein status for athletes, pregnant women, children, and seniors. With a small amount of planning, vegetarians can easily meet recommended daily protein intakes.

Fats are the third type of macronutrient. Despite their reputation, healthy fats are absolutely vital components of a balanced vegetarian diet. Essential fatty acids, including omega-3 and omega-6, promote heart health, enhance brain function, reduce inflammation, improve mood and aid absorption of important fat-soluble vitamins like A, D, E and K. Nuts, seeds and their respective butters provide unsaturated fats with omega-3s and omega-6s. Walnuts, almonds, pecans, sunflower seeds, flax seeds and hemp seeds are great choices. Avocados are another source of heart-healthy monounsaturated fats, as is olive oil. Coconuts provide medium chain saturated fats that may raise HDL, the good cholesterol.

Using oils, spreads, nuts and seeds allows vegetarians to meet daily recommendations for healthful fats.

In addition to macronutrients, vegetarian diets can amply provide all essential vitamins and minerals if thoughtfully planned. Fruits and vegetables should form the foundation of meals because their vitamin and mineral contents are immense. Leafy greens like kale, spinach and romaine lettuce are loaded with vitamins A, C, K, folate, magnesium and calcium. Winter squashes provide vitamin A and C, potassium and fiber. Berries are vitamin and antioxidant powerhouses. Bananas contain vitamin B6, potassium and magnesium. Citrus fruits like oranges and grapefruits have vitamin

C and folate. The list is extensive for produce vitamin and mineral offerings.

Additionally, many common foods are fortified to increase vegetarian intakes of key micronutrients. Cereals and grains are fortified with B vitamins including riboflavin, niacin, thiamin and folic acid. Plant milks often contain added calcium, vitamin D and B12. Meat analogues like veggie burgers and hot dogs provide iron and B12. Consuming fortified foods helps vegetarians obtain sufficient B12, iron, zinc, calcium and vitamins D and A. With care to eat across all plant food groups and select some fortified items, vegetarians can consume all the vitamins and minerals necessary for terrific health and wellbeing.

A balanced vegetarian diet can provide endless essential macro and micronutrients to fully support human health and function. With the right food choices and combinations incorporating whole plant foods, legumes, nuts, seeds, oils and fortified items, vegetarians can easily meet recommendations for carbohydrates, proteins, fats, vitamins and minerals. The vegetarian diet is nutritionally sufficient and offers immense benefits for overall wellness.

Health Benefits of a Vegetarian Diet:

In addition to their ethical and environmental merits, vegetarian diets have been associated with an array of health advantages. Studies consistently demonstrate that well-planned plant-based eating patterns correlate to reduced risk for numerous chronic diseases and conditions. Here we explore some of the top health perks linked to vegetarian diets, including benefits for heart health, weight management, diabetes prevention and cancer risk reduction.

Starting with heart health, vegetarian diets that emphasize whole foods over processed items tend to confer tremendous cardiovascular benefits. This is attributable to a number of factors. First, plant-based diets are typically lower in saturated fat and cholesterol, which supports healthy blood lipid levels. Saturated fat and cholesterol contribute to atherosclerosis, or hardening and narrowing of the arteries, by forming plaque on arterial walls. Research shows vegetarian diets improve blood lipid profiles by reducing LDL cholesterol, total cholesterol and triglyceride levels compared to non-vegetarian diets.

Vegetarians also generally have lower blood pressure levels. This is linked to increased potassium intake, reduced sodium intake, healthier body weights and higher antioxidant levels characteristic of plant-rich diets. Together, the reductions in blood cholesterol, triglycerides and blood pressure seen with vegetarian eating lower risk for heart attacks, strokes and coronary heart disease mortality. Some studies estimate vegetarians have a 32% lower risk of developing or dying from cardiovascular disease.

Beyond better blood lipids and blood pressure, vegetarian diets improve cardiovascular outcomes through other mechanisms. Fiber-rich plant foods bind to cholesterol in the gut, promoting its excretion from the body. Plant foods contain antioxidants and phytochemicals that reduce inflammation, enhance blood flow and decrease plaque buildup in arteries. Factors like lower BMI and reduced diabetes risk also indirectly improve heart health for vegetarians.

Speaking of weight management, vegetarian diets can be highly effective for achieving and maintaining healthy weights, which also supports cardiovascular wellbeing. Lower body mass indexes are consistently observed in vegetarians compared to meat eaters. One reason is the high fiber content of fruits, vegetables, whole grains and legumes, which confers a feeling of fullness. This results in less likelihood of overconsumption and better appetite control. Fiber also slows the emptying of the stomach to prolong satiety. Plant foods require more chewing time, allowing satiety signals to activate in the brain. And studies show switching to a vegetarian diet facilitates weight loss, especially visceral fat stored around the abdomen.

In addition to supporting heart health and weight management, scientific research indicates well-planned vegetarian diets can aid in the prevention and management of type 2 diabetes. Multiple studies have shown an association between plant-based eating patterns and improved blood sugar regulation, insulin sensitivity and glycemic control markers like hemoglobin A1c.

This is attributable to the high fiber and antioxidant content of vegetarian staples like beans, lentils, vegetables, fruits and whole grains. Soluble fiber delays gastric emptying and slows carbohydrate absorption from the digestive tract. This results in smaller postprandial glucose spikes and allows a gradual release of carbohydrates into the bloodstream. Fiber also reduces inflammation and oxidative stress, which are implicated in the development of insulin resistance. The collective effects of fiber translate to enhance glycemic control, decreased insulin requirements and lower risk for developing diabetes on vegetarian diets.

Beyond fiber, research indicates the protein and unsaturated fat components of plant foods improve insulin sensitivity and blood sugar management compared to animal proteins and saturated fats. For those already diagnosed with diabetes, switching to a vegetarian diet can minimize the need for medication and reduce complications of the disease.

Turning to cancer, scientific evidence indicates well-balanced vegetarian patterns may reduce risk for certain types of cancer, especially gastrointestinal cancers. Multiple aspects of plant-based diets are believed to contribute to this correlation. Firstly, vegetarians tend to consume a vast range of antioxidant and phytochemical compounds from fruits, vegetables, nuts, seeds, beans and whole grains. These agents have favorable effects on cell signaling pathways involved in cancer progression, prompting apoptosis of malignant cells and inhibiting tumor growth.

Additionally, the fiber content of plant foods supports healthy gut microbiota. Research shows gut bacteria metabolize bile acids and estrogens in ways that lower colon cancer risk in those consuming plant-based diets. The high fiber content also dilutes potential carcinogens and pro-inflammatory factors in the gut, while promoting regular bowel movements to promptly eliminate waste and toxins.

However, it should be noted that individual dietary choices like consuming adequate fruits and vegetables versus overly refined carbs impact cancer risk as much as simply adhering to a vegetarian diet. Lifestyle factors beyond diet are also hugely influential, including smoking, sun exposure, alcohol intake and exercise habits. So while vegetarian diets show promise for cancer prevention, they should be evaluated in context of the overall eating pattern and other lifestyle factors.

Science clearly demonstrates the myriad benefits of vegetarian diets for health promotion and chronic disease risk reduction. Reduced risk of heart disease, improvements in weight management, enhanced diabetes prevention and possible protective advantages against some cancers are well documented in vegetarians compared to non-vegetarians. Of course, exercise, sleep, stress levels and other lifestyle variables significantly contribute to overall health. But when paired with other healthy behaviors, a well-balanced vegetarian diet can be a cornerstone of good health.

Addressing Nutritional Concerns:

When considering a vegetarian diet, many have concerns about meeting nutrient needs without animal products. However, with intentional meal planning and variety, vegetarians can easily consume adequate protein, vitamins, minerals, and essential fatty acids for optimal health. This requires an understanding of key nutrients of concern and incorporation of the best plant-based sources.

Starting with protein, this macronutrient is vital for building, repairing and maintaining tissues and cells. Protein is comprised of amino acids, some of which the body can synthesize while others called essential amino acids must come from food. Animal products contain all essential amino acids, leading to a misconception that plant proteins are incomplete. However, by consuming a variety of plant-based protein sources over a day, vegetarians can readily meet needs.

Options like legumes, whole grains, nuts and seeds all contribute different amino acid profiles that complement each other. Beans, lentils and peas are packed with around 15 grams protein per cooked cup. Ancient grains like quinoa and amaranth contain approximately 8 grams per cooked cup, as do nuts and seeds. Soy foods like tofu, tempeh and edamame are vegetarian protein powerhouses, providing a full array of essential amino acids. Even produce like spinach, artichokes, broccoli and potatoes contribute small amounts of protein that add up. With balanced meal planning, vegetarians can easily achieve recommended daily intakes of this crucial macronutrient.

In terms of micronutrients, attention to a few key vitamins and minerals is prudent to ensure vegetarians meet needs. For iron, beans, lentils, spinach, nuts and seeds are rich sources. Pairing these iron-rich foods with vitamin C-containing foods enhances absorption, as the acidity increases iron's bioavailability. So enjoying beans over a bed of greens or lemon-dressed lentils salad aids iron intake.

Calcium is another mineral of import. Leafy greens like spinach and kale, tofu, almonds, figs and sesame seeds supply ample calcium. Fortified plant milks and juices also boost vegetarian calcium levels. Magnesium supports calcium absorption, so consuming whole grains, nuts and legumes high in this mineral optimizes calcium status.

Vitamin B12 deserves consideration since it is primarily obtained from animal products. Vegetarians should consume fortified foods like non-dairy milk and breakfast cereal or take a supplement. Nutritional yeast is another option. Due to poor absorption, vitamin B12 from plant sources alone may be insufficient, warranting fortified foods or a supplement.

Lastly, essential fatty acids like omega-3s are crucial for vegans. Alpha-linoleic acid or ALA is the plant-based omega-3 found in walnuts, flaxseeds, chia seeds and hemp seeds. Some converts to EPA and DHA to support cardiovascular and brain function. However, this conversion can be inefficient. Using ground flax or chia seeds, walnut oil and seaweed provide ALA while also considering an algae-based omega-3 supplement to enhance EPA and DHA status.

When thoughtfully planned, vegetarian diets can provide endless essential macro and micronutrients for outstanding health and performance. Focusing on whole, minimally processed plant staples like beans, lentils, nuts, seeds, whole grains, fruits, vegetables oils and fortified foods ensures nutrient needs are met. If any concerns arise around potential deficiencies, supplements offer an insurance policy. With awareness of key nutrients and strategic meal planning, vegetarians can thrive while eating an exclusively plant-based diet.

When adopting a vegetarian diet, it is understandable to have concerns about meeting nutrient needs without consuming animal products. However, with careful planning and intentionality, vegetarians can readily satisfy daily recommended intakes of all essential vitamins, minerals and other micronutrients critical for optimal health and functioning. Here are some tips and wisdom for vegetarians looking to ensure a well-balanced, nutritionally-adequate diet:

First and foremost, variety and diversity are paramount. Include a wide range of plant-based foods across all food groups - grains, legumes, nuts, seeds, vegetables, fruits, oils. No single plant item contains every essential nutrient, so eating a spectrum of produce, whole grains, beans, lentils, nuts and seeds is key. This mix maximizes the likelihood of covering nutritional bases and allows complementary pairings that provide complete proteins.

Whole grains deserve particular focus as nutrient-dense carbohydrate staples of a vegetarian diet. Options like quinoa, amaranth, buckwheat, oats, brown rice, farro and whole grain barley, breads and pastas provide an array of vitamins, minerals, protein and fiber. Go for whole grains over refined grains whenever possible. And pair grains with beans or lentils to make complete proteins.

Speaking of protein, consuming a variety of plant-based protein sources ensures adequate amino acid intake. Legumes like beans, peas and lentils are protein all-stars. Lesser known options like tempeh and Ezekiel bread also contribute. Nuts, seeds, tofu and vegetarian meat substitutes like seitan boost protein content. Even many vegetables and ancient grains contain modest protein levels that add up over the day.

Healthy fats also deserve attention to meet omega essential fatty acid needs. Nuts, seeds and derived butters provide anti-inflammatory omega-3 fats. Avocados supply monounsaturated fats that support heart health. Olive, canola and coconut oil deliver beneficial fats for brain functioning and vitamin absorption. Avoid saturated fats from processed and fried foods.

In terms of micronutrients, dark leafy greens are nutritional rockstars, packed with vitamins A, C, K, B9, magnesium, potassium and more. Broccoli, brussels sprouts, peppers and carrots are also nutrient-dense choices. Berries overflow with antioxidants and phytochemicals that promote health and longevity. Slowly eating nuts and seeds maximizes absorption of their vitamins, minerals and healthy fats.

Specific nutrients like calcium, iron, zinc, vitamin D, vitamin B12 and omega-3s may need particular attention. Fortified foods like plant milks, breakfast cereals and meat alternatives boost intake of these critical nutrients. Calcium-set tofu, zinc-rich pumpkin seeds, iron-laden spinach and lentils are examples of selective foods to emphasize.

Additionally, some vegetarians may benefit from supplements to fill potential gaps. A regular, well-absorbed vitamin B12 supplement is commonly advised since this vitamin is scarce in plant foods. Similarly, a microalgae omega-3 supplement enhances DHA and EPA status. Multivitamins or targeted zinc, iron, calcium and vitamin D supplements can provide a nutritional safety net as needed.

With diligence to eat an array of minimally processed plant foods, attention to key nutrient sources like whole grains, legumes, nuts and seeds, selective use of fortified and supplemented items, and balance across all food groups, vegetarians can readily meet and exceed all nutritional requirements. Variety and balance centered on whole plant foods, along with strategic supplementation, ensures vegetarians thrive on a diet free of animal products.

Protein Sources

Protein is an essential macronutrient for building muscle, supporting immune function, creating enzymes and promoting overall health. Traditionally, meat and other animal products were considered superior protein sources due to their complete amino acid profiles. However, a variety of plant-based foods can readily meet protein needs for vegetarians and vegans. Consuming a diverse array of plant proteins ensures adequate intake of all the essential amino acids required for optimal functioning.

Legumes including beans, lentils, peas and peanuts are stellar protein providers, with around 15 grams per cooked cup. Kidney beans, black beans, chickpeas, soybeans and green peas are loaded with protein. Lentils come in red, brown, black, green and other varieties, all providing substantial protein. These legumes also supply ample fiber, vitamins and minerals like iron, zinc and magnesium.

Nuts and seeds are another category of plant proteins. Almonds, pistachios, walnuts, cashews, pumpkin seeds and sunflower seeds range from 5-7 grams protein per ounce. Nut and seed butters retain the protein content in a spreadable form. Hemp seeds offer over 10 grams protein per ounce. Flax, chia and hemp seeds also provide anti-inflammatory omega-3 fats. The protein, fiber and healthy fats in nuts and seeds aid satiety as well.

Grains like quinoa, amaranth, buckwheat and oats also contribute modest levels of high quality protein. Quinoa leads the way with 8 grams per cooked cup. Quinoa and amaranth are unique whole grains that contain complete proteins with all nine essential amino acids.

Pairing grains with legumes provides a well-rounded amino acid profile.

Tofu, tempeh, edamame and other soy-based foods are complete vegetarian proteins. Half a cup of tofu contains around 10 grams of protein and also provides calcium, iron and antioxidants. Tempeh, miso, natto and soy milk similarly provide solid protein content. Edamame are immature soybeans that make a protein-rich snack.

For vegetarians who consume dairy, Greek yogurt, cheese and cottage cheese offer ample protein. Six ounces of Greek yogurt contributes 15-20 grams, surpassing the protein in regular yogurt. Cheese, milk and yogurt provide calcium and vitamin D as well.

Vegetarians can also get protein from unexpected sources like seitan, nutritional yeast, vegetables, Ezekiel bread and pasta, milk alternatives and protein powders. Seitan, made from wheat gluten, contains about 25 grams protein per serving. Nutritional yeast is fortified with vitamin B12 and packs 8 grams protein per two tablespoons. Green vegetables have small amounts of protein that add up, with spinach at 5 grams per cooked cup. Most breads, plant milks, pasta and meat substitutes contain at least a few grams of protein too. Protein supplements derived from plants like peas, rice and hemp help meet needs.

To ensure adequate essential amino acid intake, vegetarians should aim to incorporate a variety of these plant-based protein sources into a day's meals. Consuming complementary proteins together, such as rice and beans or hummus on whole grain toast, can yield a complete protein profile. Including proteins like soy, quinoa or nutritional yeast improves essential amino acid intake as well. A balanced plate containing grains, legumes, nuts, seeds, vegetables and soy covers all the protein bases. With planning, vegetarians can easily meet and even exceed their daily protein requirements from plant sources alone.

The significance of vitamin and mineral intake for vegetarians and vegans

A nutritious vegetarian or vegan diet can readily provide all the essential vitamins, minerals and other micronutrients required for optimal health. However, certain nutrients deserve special attention and planning in plant-based diets to ensure adequate intake. Being mindful of key micronutrients and the best dietary sources allows vegetarians to reap the many benefits of eating plant-based while meeting all nutritional needs.

Starting with minerals, iron is essential for producing hemoglobin to transport oxygen throughout the body. Plant sources like lentils, beans, spinach and broccoli contain non-heme iron that isn't absorbed as well as iron from meat. Combining vitamin C-rich foods like oranges, peppers or strawberries with iron-rich foods enhances absorption, as vitamin C's acidity helps convert iron into an absorbable form. Dark leafy greens offer both iron and vitamin C for optimal intake. Iron-fortified cereals and breads also boost levels.

Another mineral, calcium, is crucial for proper muscle and nerve functioning and building strong bones. Leafy greens - kale, collards, broccoli and bok choy - are excellent plant-based sources. Almonds, oranges, figs, beans, tofu cooked with calcium, and sesame seeds and tahini also provide calcium. Likewise, consuming plant milks fortified with calcium assists in meeting needs. The vitamin D status affects calcium levels, so adequate sun exposure, fortified foods and supplementation may be necessary to support bone health.

In terms of vitamins, vitamin B12 requires attention in plant-based diets, as it is predominantly found in animal products. Vegans and vegetarians need vitamin B12-fortified items like plant milks, nutritional yeast, cereals or egg substitutes. Those avoiding fortified foods will likely require B12 supplements or injections to prevent deficiency. Proper vitamin B12 status is crucial for neurological function and red blood cell formation.

Another vitamin, vitamin A, supports immune function and vision. Alpha-carotene found in carrots, sweet potatoes and greens can be converted to active vitamin A, though less efficiently than animal sources like liver. Therefore, vegetarians may need more dietary or supplemental vitamin A to meet needs. Vitamin D also boosts immunity and aids calcium absorption. Sunlight enables vitamin D synthesis in skin, but cloudy climates and indoor lifestyles may necessitate fortified milks and cereals or supplements.

In addition to vitamins and minerals, omega-3 fatty acids EPA and DHA support cognitive and heart health. Vegetarian sources like walnuts, flax and chia seeds provide ALA that partially converts to EPA and DHA. However, a direct microalgae oil supplement maximizes omega-3 status. Probiotic foods can also enhance mineral absorption, particularly for iron and calcium.

Beyond these highlighted nutrients, eating an array of whole plant foods like vegetables, fruits, beans, lentils, nuts, seeds and grains provides a spectrum of beneficial micronutrients. Antioxidants in colorful produce defend against chronic disease. Fibrous fruits, vegetables and whole grains promote healthy cholesterol, blood sugar and weight. With attention to key nutrient sources and selective supplementation, vegetarians can consume plentiful essential vitamins and minerals for terrific wellbeing.

Chapter Three

Equipment

In the past decade, vegetarian diets have soared in popularity for an array of reasons spanning health, ethics and environmentalism. With this expansion, the demand for specialized equipment to maximize the culinary potential of plant-based cooking has also grown. While basic tools allow preparing simple meatless meals, upgrading to high-quality vegetarian-specific appliances and gadgets can truly elevate the cuisine to new heights. Investing in the optimal kitchen tools provides creative freedom to fully explore the diverse ingredients and techniques of vegetarian fare.

For starters, a powerful blender opens up endless possibilities for making velvety plant-based smoothies, soups, nut milks, sauces, dressings and more. Blenders like Vitamix or Blendtec have commercial grade motors to puree the toughest whole foods like kale, frozen produce and nuts into utterly smooth creations. Their speed and blade power far surpass regular blenders, ensuring smooth results without annoying chunks. This allows whipping up incredible blended items like creamy carrot ginger soup, strawberry banana smoothies, homemade almond milk and savory cashew cream sauces.

Multi-function cookers like Instant Pots also prove invaluable for meatless cooking by serving as a pressure cooker, slow cooker, rice maker and more. Their pressure cooking settings quickly tenderize beans, tough veggies like beets, and accelerate cooking times for soups and stews. Meanwhile, their slow cook function allows waking up to ready vegetarian chili, oatmeal or curries. This versatility streamlines weeknight vegetarian meals and reduces appliance clutter.

When it comes to actual cooking, quality pots and pans suited for plant-based diets make all the difference. Non-stick ceramic or hard anodized cookware allows sautéing and stir-frying delicate tofu, tempeh and vegetables without sticking. Saucepots with steamer baskets enable simultaneous steaming of veggies and grains. Sturdy Dutch ovens work wonderfully for vegetarian soups, stews, chili and one-pot meals. Investing in durable, non-stick, dishwasher safe cookware simplifies preparing all kinds of vegetarian dishes.

Vegetable spiralizers allow creating low-carb veggie noodles from zucchini, carrots, beets and other produce in mere minutes. Models like the Paderno, Veggetti or Spiralizer Tri-Blade attach to kitchen counters, while handheld spiralizers offer portability. They open infinite options for healthy vegetarian "pastas" and noodle replacements. Zucchini noodles with pesto or carrot noodles with ginger-miso dressing become gourmet, plant-based meals thanks to this gadget.

Food processors like Cuisinart make easy work of numerous vegetarian prep tasks like chopping nuts, blending pesto, grating cheese, slicing veggies, shredding lettuce and crafting veggie burgers or fritters. Their slicing and grating discs minimize prep time while offering consistency. Meal prepping chopped vegetables and shredded cheese for the week has never been simpler.

Cast iron skillets have unparalleled heat retention perfect for getting a sear on tofu, tempeh, portobellos or roasted vegetables. Modern vegetable peelers, graters, colanders and cutting boards in bright colors also inspire meal prepping. And silicone mats enable roasting vegetables without sticking or pans.

While basic tools work for simple dishes, upgrading to these game-changing appliances and gadgets elevates vegetarian cuisine to new levels. Blending, steaming, spiralizing and pressure cooking become one-touch affairs. Non-stick cookware prevents delicately sticking. Food processors decrease chopping time. Quality kitchen equipment unleashes creativity and possibilities for home chefs seeking to prepare exceptional plant-based meals. The investment pays dividends in terms of saved time, reduced frustration and increased culinary enjoyment. For devoted vegetarian home cooks, outfitting the kitchen with high-performance tools is absolutely worthwhile.

Importance of having the right kitchen equipment

Having the proper tools and ingredients on hand is essential for preparing delicious and nutritious vegetarian meals on a consistent basis. When first transitioning to a vegetarian diet, many find themselves relying too heavily on easy-to-make foods like pasta or frozen meals. While these can be part of a healthy diet, vegetarians will benefit greatly from equipping their kitchen for more variety. Below are some key equipment and pantry items to have on hand, as well as tips for building skills and meal plans.

Equipment:

The foundation of any kitchen is having high quality pots, pans, baking sheets and utensils. Stainless steel, ceramic and cast iron are all good options. Make sure to have a range of sizes for boiling pasta, sautéing vegetables, making soups and more. A sturdy set of knives is also essential, along with a cutting board, peeler, grater and colander. Appliance-wise, a blender or food processor is invaluable for making hummus, pizza dough, veggie burgers and other staples. An immersion blender is great for pureeing soups right in the pot. A microwave or toaster oven are convenient for quickly heating leftovers.

Pantry:

A well-stocked pantry ensures you always have key ingredients on hand for impromptu meals. Shelf-stable proteins like beans, lentils, nuts and seeds enable endless meal options. Canned or dry varieties like chickpeas, black beans and edamame are low cost and easy to incorporate. Nut butters, hemp seeds and quinoa also pack a protein punch. For produce, keep potatoes, sweet potatoes, onions and garlic stocked. Other staples include broth, oil, vinegars, spices, herbs, flour, pasta and rice.

Don't forget flavor boosters like tamari or soy sauce, tahini, salsa and nutritional yeast. Canned goods like tomatoes, coconut milk and vegetables make assembling dishes quick and simple. Dried fruit, eggs, plant-based milk and cheese are also good to have around. Take stock of what you use regularly and create a list for easy shopping.

Skills:

The magic truly happens when you have the right tools and ingredients for recipes that excite you. Take inventory of current skills in the kitchen. Are there vegetarian dishes you love to make and want to perfect? Look up new ways to prepare your favorite vegetables.

Challenge yourself to try globally-inspired cuisines that tantalize your tastebuds.

Follow vegetarian chefs and food blogs that offer lessons for building knife skills, cooking grains and beans from scratch, and blending balanced meals. Getting comfortable with cooking techniques like sautéing, steaming, braising and roasting expands your versatility. Don't be afraid to experiment and get creative! Soon your enhanced skills turn basic ingredients into satisfying meals.

Planning:

Finally, having a plan sets you up for success, especially for busy weeks. Take time on the weekend to browse recipes, write a grocery list and prep ingredients. Cook a big batch of grains or beans to use throughout the week. Chop vegetables for easy cooking or have them ready for snacks.

Invest in food storage like mason jars and reusable containers. Prepare make-ahead staples like a veggie chili, lentil soup or breakfast bake. Having meal components ready to assemble saves time and energy. It also prevents takeout temptations after long days. Prior planning translates to more homecooked and healthier meals.

Equipping your kitchen and cultivating skills for vegetarian cooking may feel daunting at first. But having the right tools and ingredients at your fingertips, along with go-to recipes, makes meal prep joyful and sustainable. A well-stocked kitchen guarantees you always have quick and nourishing plant-based options. With practice, you'll gain versatility in the kitchen for crafting delicious vegetarian meals full of variety and flavor.

How proper tools and ingredients can make cooking more efficient and enjoyable.

Emphasizing the importance of proper tools and ingredients in cooking is essential because they play a significant role in making the culinary experience efficient, enjoyable, and ultimately successful. From enabling smoother cooking processes to enhancing the flavors and textures of dishes, the right tools and ingredients can transform a meal from ordinary to extraordinary. Here's a detailed discussion on how proper tools and ingredients contribute to efficient and enjoyable cooking:

1. Efficiency in Cooking:

Time-Saving: The right tools can significantly reduce prep time. Sharp knives, efficient peelers, and versatile gadgets can streamline chopping, slicing, and dicing tasks, allowing you to prepare ingredients quickly and efficiently.

Consistency: Proper tools ensure uniformity in cutting and chopping, leading to even cooking and better presentation. This is crucial, especially when working with ingredients that require consistent sizes, such as vegetables for stir-fries or fruits for desserts.

Multi-Tasking: Many kitchen tools are designed to perform multiple tasks, which can simplify complex recipes. For instance, a food processor can chop, blend, and knead, eliminating the need for separate gadgets.

Precision: Accurate measuring tools ensure you're using the right proportions of ingredients, which is crucial for achieving desired flavors and textures. Baking, for example, relies heavily on precise measurements.

2. Enhancing Flavors and Textures:

Ingredients' Quality: Using high-quality ingredients, such as fresh produce and premium spices, can significantly impact the final dish's flavor profile. Fresh herbs, aromatic spices, and quality oils can elevate even simple dishes.

Texture Mastery: Proper tools can help achieve desired textures. Blenders and food processors can create smooth sauces and creamy soups, while graters and zesters add delightful textures to salads and desserts.

Flavor Infusion: Certain tools, like mortar and pestle, can release oils and compounds from herbs and spices, intensifying their flavors and aromas. This can be particularly beneficial in creating robust marinades and dressings.

3. Creative Freedom and Enjoyment:

Experimentation: The right tools and ingredients empower you to experiment with new recipes and cuisines. A well-stocked pantry allows you to explore diverse flavors and techniques without constant trips to the grocery store.

Culinary Confidence: Proper tools make cooking tasks feel less daunting. Knowing you have the necessary equipment gives you the confidence to take on more challenging recipes and techniques.

Culinary Artistry: Cooking becomes a form of creative expression when you have the tools to transform raw ingredients into visually appealing and flavorful dishes. Presentation tools, such as piping bags and molds, enable artistic plating.

4. Reduced Stress and Increased Enjoyment:

Stress Reduction: Having the right tools can reduce stress in the kitchen. When you're well-equipped, you're less likely to encounter unexpected challenges during the cooking process.

Smooth Execution: Cooking becomes more enjoyable when you can smoothly execute recipes without interruptions caused by missing tools or ingredients.

Family and Social Time: Efficient cooking allows you to spend more quality time with family and friends. Instead of spending hours in the kitchen, you can prepare meals efficiently and join the gathering.

Must-have kitchen tools

In the realm of vegetarian cooking, having the right kitchen tools can be the key to transforming fresh produce and plant-based ingredients into delicious, wholesome meals. From the precise art of chopping vegetables to the creation of creamy sauces and soups, each tool serves a unique purpose in the vegetarian kitchen. In this discussion, we'll explore the essential kitchen tools that every vegetarian cook should have in their culinary arsenal.

1. Knives: Different Types and Their Uses

Knives are the backbone of any kitchen, and for vegetarian cooking, they are indispensable. Different types of knives serve various purposes, ensuring efficient preparation of vegetables, fruits, and other ingredients:

Chef's Knife: This versatile, all-purpose knife is a must-have. It's ideal for chopping, dicing, and slicing a wide range of ingredients, from hearty vegetables like potatoes to delicate herbs.

Paring Knife: With a small, narrow blade, a paring knife is perfect for precise tasks such as peeling and trimming.

Serrated Knife: Known for its jagged edge, a serrated knife is essential for cutting through foods with tough exteriors and soft interiors, like tomatoes and bread.

Utility Knife: This knife bridges the gap between a chef's knife and a paring knife. It's great for tasks that are too small for a chef's knife but too big for a paring knife.

2. Cutting Boards, Mixing Bowls, Measuring Cups, and Spoons

These foundational tools contribute to an organized and efficient cooking process:

Cutting Boards: Invest in high-quality, durable cutting boards. Having multiple boards can prevent cross-contamination when working with different ingredients.

Mixing Bowls: A variety of sizes allows for easy mixing of ingredients, from tossing salads to mixing dough for baking.

Measuring Cups and Spoons: Accurate measurements are crucial for consistent results, especially in baking. Both liquid and dry ingredient measurements should be covered.

3. Pots and Pans Suitable for Vegetarian Cooking

Skillet: A good skillet or frying pan is essential for sautéing vegetables, making stir-fries, and cooking pancakes. Opt for one with a non-stick surface for easier clean-up.

Saucepan: This versatile pot is perfect for cooking sauces, gravies, and soups. It comes in various sizes, allowing you to choose the right one for the quantity of food you're preparing.

Stockpot: When making large batches of soups, stews, or pasta, a stockpot is a must. Its ample capacity and tall sides accommodate a wide range of dishes.

4. Baking Essentials: Baking Sheets, Muffin Tins, and Cake Pans

Baking Sheets: These flat sheets are perfect for roasting vegetables, baking cookies, and making sheet pan dinners. Opt for ones with a rim to prevent spillage.

Muffin Tins: Useful for baking muffins and cupcakes, but also great for making mini quiches, frittatas, and other single-serving dishes.

Cake Pans: Necessary for baking cakes and other baked desserts. Choose from various shapes and sizes to suit your needs.

5. Blenders, Food Processors, and Immersion Blenders

Blenders: Blenders are essential for making smoothies, sauces, and creamy soups. High-speed blenders are particularly effective in breaking down fibrous vegetables and fruits.

Food Processors: These versatile machines can chop, slice, dice, and even knead dough. They're invaluable for preparing ingredients like breadcrumbs, nut butters, and pesto.

Immersion Blenders: Also known as stick blenders, these are perfect for blending soups and sauces directly in the pot, eliminating the need for transferring hot liquids.

6. Oven and Stovetop Considerations for Various Cooking Techniques

Oven: Ovens are crucial for baking, roasting, and broiling. They allow you to create a wide range of dishes, from casseroles to roasted vegetables.

Stovetop: A versatile stovetop with multiple burners enables you to simultaneously cook various components of a meal. Different heat levels are essential for different cooking techniques, such as sautéing, simmering, and boiling.

Grill Pan: While not a substitute for an outdoor grill, a grill pan can add charred marks and smoky flavors to vegetables and other ingredients.

Equipment that can enhance vegetarian cooking experiences

Vegetarian cooking is a journey of creativity and innovation, and having the right tools can significantly enhance this culinary experience. Beyond the basic kitchen essentials, specialized equipment can elevate your vegetarian dishes to new heights. From turning vegetables into innovative noodles to streamlining ingredient preparation and protein handling, each tool serves a unique purpose. In this discussion, we'll delve into the specialized equipment that can enrich your vegetarian cooking adventures.

1. Spiralizers for Making Vegetable Noodles:

Spiralizers are game-changers for introducing variety and vibrancy to vegetarian meals. These tools transform vegetables like zucchini, carrots, and sweet potatoes into delightful noodle-like strands, offering a healthier alternative to traditional pasta. Vegetable noodles not only add texture but also increase your intake of nutrient-rich veggies. With spiralizers, you can create visually appealing dishes like zucchini "spaghetti," carrot "linguine," and sweet potato "fettuccine." These innovative presentations not only please the eyes but also contribute to a more nutritious and exciting meal.

2. Vegetable Peelers and Corers for Precise Prep:

Vegetable peelers and corers might seem basic, but their precision and efficiency are invaluable for vegetarian cooking. A good vegetable peeler ensures you can quickly remove skins, enhancing the aesthetic appeal and texture of your dishes. Corers are particularly handy for tasks like removing apple cores or prepping bell peppers for stuffing. Precise preparation ensures even cooking and better integration of flavors, making your vegetarian creations more enjoyable.

3. Salad Spinners and Herb Strippers for Efficient Ingredient Handling:

Salads and fresh herbs are staples in vegetarian cuisine, and specialized tools like salad spinners and herb strippers streamline their preparation:

Salad Spinners: These tools remove excess water from washed greens, preventing soggy salads. Dry greens not only contribute to a better eating experience but also allow dressings to adhere more effectively.

Herb Strippers: Herb strippers efficiently remove leaves from herb stems, saving time and effort when preparing ingredients like basil, cilantro, and parsley. This ensures that only the flavorful leaves are used, reducing waste and enhancing the taste of your dishes.

4. Tofu Presses and Nut Milk Bags for Plant-Based Protein Preparation:

For vegetarians, plant-based protein sources like tofu and nut milk are essential components of their diet. Specialized equipment makes their preparation more efficient and yields better results:

Tofu Presses: Tofu presses remove excess moisture from tofu, allowing it to absorb flavors and marinades more effectively. This leads to tastier and more textured tofu dishes, whether you're making stir-fries, curries, or even vegan desserts.

Nut Milk Bags: Nut milk bags are indispensable for making homemade nut milks and plant-based yogurt. These bags effectively strain out solids, yielding creamy, smooth, and flavorful results without the need for commercial additives.

5. Rice Cookers and Slow Cookers for Easy One-Pot Meals:

Rice cookers and slow cookers are versatile kitchen appliances that simplify vegetarian cooking:

Rice Cookers: While primarily designed for cooking rice, modern rice cookers can do much more. They can prepare a variety of grains, steam vegetables, and even create one-pot rice cooker meals that incorporate veggies, beans, and spices.

Slow Cookers: Slow cookers are a boon for busy individuals who want hearty, comforting meals without constant supervision. They're perfect for simmering soups, stews, chili, and other dishes, allowing flavors to meld while you go about your day.

6. Dehydrators for Making Snacks and Dried Ingredients:

Dehydrators are ideal for preserving the flavors and nutrients of fruits, vegetables, and herbs:

Snacks: Dehydrators let you create wholesome snacks like fruit chips, kale chips, and even dried veggie jerky. These snacks are not only convenient but also free from additives commonly found in store-bought alternatives.

Dried Ingredients: Dehydrators are also handy for drying herbs, making your own dried tomatoes, and preserving excess produce.

Dried ingredients can be used in various dishes to add depth of flavor.

Specialized equipment has the power to transform your vegetarian cooking experiences. From enhancing the visual appeal of your dishes to streamlining ingredient preparation and protein handling, each tool serves a unique purpose in the vegetarian kitchen. By incorporating these tools into your culinary repertoire, you can explore new textures, flavors, and cooking techniques that elevate your vegetarian creations to new dimensions. Whether you're making vegetable noodles, creamy nut milks, or vibrant salads, specialized equipment empowers you to unleash your creativity and embark on a flavorful journey in the world of vegetarian cuisine.

Stocking a Vegetarian Pantry

A well-stocked pantry is the backbone of any successful kitchen, and for vegetarians, it's the foundation for crafting diverse, flavorful, and nutrient-rich meals. From grains and legumes to spices and dairy alternatives, having a variety of staple ingredients at your disposal empowers you to create delicious vegetarian dishes without constant trips to the grocery store. In this discussion, we'll explore a comprehensive list of essential pantry items every vegetarian kitchen should have.

1. Grains: Rice, Quinoa, Pasta, Oats, and More

Grains serve as the base for many vegetarian meals, providing energy, fiber, and essential nutrients:

Rice: Both white and brown rice are versatile staples. Brown rice offers more fiber and nutrients, while white rice has a lighter texture.

Quinoa: A complete protein source, quinoa is rich in fiber and essential amino acids. It can be used in salads, bowls, and even as a breakfast option.

Pasta: Choose whole grain or legume-based pasta for added nutrition. Pasta dishes are endlessly customizable with various sauces and vegetables.

Oats: Perfect for breakfast, oats can be turned into oatmeal, granola, or added to smoothies for a nutritional boost.

Whole Wheat Flour: A versatile baking staple that can also be used to make flatbreads and homemade tortillas.

2. Legumes: Lentils, Beans, Chickpeas, and More

Legumes are rich in plant-based protein, fiber, and various nutrients:

Lentils: Red, green, and brown lentils are versatile and cook quickly. They're perfect for soups, stews, and curries.

Beans: Varieties like black beans, kidney beans, and pinto beans can be used in salads, dips, burritos, and more.

Chickpeas: Also known as garbanzo beans, chickpeas are essential for making hummus, curries, and crispy chickpea snacks.

Lentil Pasta: An excellent gluten-free alternative to traditional pasta, lentil pasta is higher in protein and fiber.

3. Canned Goods: Tomatoes, Coconut Milk, Vegetable Broth, etc.

Canned goods provide convenience and flavor to vegetarian cooking:

Canned Tomatoes: Crushed, diced, or whole tomatoes are the base for many sauces, soups, and stews.

Coconut Milk: Used in a variety of savory and sweet dishes, coconut milk adds creaminess and flavor.

Vegetable Broth: A versatile ingredient for soups, risottos, and sauces. Opt for low-sodium options for more control over the salt content.

4. Baking Essentials: Flour, Sugar, Baking Powder, etc.

Baking essentials are crucial for creating a variety of baked goods:

Flour: Beyond whole wheat flour, all-purpose and alternative flours like almond and coconut are versatile for baking.

Sugar: White, brown, and natural sweeteners like maple syrup and agave nectar are useful for baking and cooking.

Baking Powder and Baking Soda: These leavening agents are essential for making baked goods rise.

5. Oils and Vinegars: Olive Oil, Coconut Oil, Balsamic Vinegar, etc.

Oils and vinegars are the foundation of many dressings and cooking methods:

Olive Oil: A heart-healthy oil suitable for sautéing, roasting, and making dressings.

Coconut Oil: Ideal for baking and high-heat cooking, coconut oil adds a unique flavor to dishes.

Balsamic Vinegar: Adds depth and tang to salads and marinades.

6. Spices and Herbs: Basics like Salt and Pepper, Plus a Variety of Seasonings

Spices and herbs are the flavor enhancers that bring vegetarian dishes to life:

Salt and Pepper: Basic seasonings that form the foundation of flavor in most dishes.

Cumin, Paprika, and Chili Powder: Adds warmth and depth to dishes like curries and chili.

Turmeric: Known for its anti-inflammatory properties and vibrant color, it's a staple in curries and rice dishes.

Basil, Thyme, Rosemary, and Oregano: A variety of dried and fresh herbs add complexity to dishes.

7. Nuts and Seeds: Almonds, Walnuts, Chia Seeds, etc.

Nuts and seeds provide crunch, healthy fats, and essential nutrients:

Almonds: Great for snacking, adding to salads, or making almond butter.

Walnuts: A good source of omega-3 fatty acids, walnuts can be added to oatmeal, baked goods, and salads.

Chia Seeds: Rich in fiber and omega-3s, chia seeds can be used to make chia pudding, smoothies, and as an egg substitute in baking.

8. Sauces and Condiments: Soy Sauce, Tahini, Hot Sauce, etc.

Sauces and condiments add depth and complexity to vegetarian dishes:

Soy Sauce or Tamari: Essential for savory dishes and stir-fries.

Tahini: Used in Middle Eastern cuisine and dressings, tahini adds creaminess and nuttiness.

Hot Sauce: Adds heat and flavor to various dishes, from tacos to tofu scrambles.

9. Dairy Alternatives: Non-Dairy Milk, Yogurt, and Vegan Cheese

Dairy alternatives are essential for creating creamy textures in vegan recipes:

Non-Dairy Milk: Almond, soy, coconut, and oat milk are versatile substitutes for cow's milk.

Non-Dairy Yogurt: Coconut, almond, and soy-based yogurts are excellent for parfaits, smoothies, and baking.

Vegan Cheese: Available in various flavors and styles, vegan cheese adds a satisfying cheesy element to dishes.

10. Sweeteners: Maple Syrup, Agave Nectar, etc.

Sweeteners provide a touch of sweetness to both sweet and savory dishes:

Maple Syrup and Agave Nectar: Natural sweeteners for drizzling on pancakes, oatmeal, and desserts.

11. Fresh Produce: Refrigerator Essentials like Onions, Garlic, and Lemons

Fresh produce forms the core of vegetarian cooking:

Onions and Garlic: These aromatic staples are the base for countless dishes and add depth to flavors.

Lemons: Used for their zest and juice, lemons brighten up dishes, dressings, and marinades.

A well-rounded pantry is a vegetarian cook's best friend. It enables you to craft an array of dishes with depth, flavor, and nutrition. From grains and legumes to spices, oils, and dairy alternatives, these staple ingredients form the canvas upon which you paint your culinary creations. With a well-stocked pantry, you're empowered to explore the world of vegetarian cuisine, experiment with flavors, and enjoy a diverse range of nutritious and delicious meals.

Organizing Your Pantry

A well-organized vegetarian pantry is the secret to easy, healthy plant-based cooking. With the right ingredients and equipment on hand, you can quickly assemble delicious meals any day of the week. Follow these tips to maximize space, keep items fresh, and know exactly where to find what you need.

Categorize:

The first step is sorting all items into logical categories. Group like items together such as all canned goods on one shelf, baking supplies on another. You may sort by type of ingredients or frequency of use. Other handy categories include snacks, oils and condiments, spices and dry goods.

Label clearly:

Once organized into categories, use labels to identify what belongs where. Masking tape, sticky notes or chalkboard labels work great.

This prevents that frenzied searching when you need an ingredient for a recipe. You'll save time knowing exactly where everything is at a glance.

Use containers:

Use containers of different sizes to hold bulk items like rice, quinoa, beans and more. Clear containers allow you to see contents. Measure and label the volume on the lid for easy scooping. Uniform containers keep the space neat and make inventory simpler. Invest in airtight containers to keep items like flour, sugar and cereal fresh.

Store wisely:

Be smart about where and how you store certain items. Keep beans, nuts, seeds, flours and grains in a cool, dark space to prevent spoilage. Storing canned goods and boxed items on shelves makes them visible and reachable. Use lazy susans or tiered racks to better access items in the back. The top shelves can hold lesser used items or appliances. Place everyday cooking essentials at eye level for convenience.

Fridge organization:

Apply these same principles inside your refrigerator. Store produce in clear crisp drawers to easily spot what needs using. Have a dedicated shelf for condiments, sauces and dressings. Use the door for items you frequently grab like non-dairy milk and butter. Place leftovers in clear glass containers labeled with dates. Regularly check for expired items.

Meal planning:

An organized pantry lends itself to smarter weekly meal plans. You can quickly glance at current inventory and plan recipes accordingly. Make a list to use up soon-to-expire items first. Meal planning also helps identify staples running low so you remember to restock. An organized pantry prevents buying duplicate ingredients.

Pantry staples:

A vegetarian pantry should be stocked with nutrient-dense, versatile ingredients full of flavor. Prioritize plant-based proteins like beans, lentils, nuts, seeds and tofu. Include ancient grains, sprouted breads and alternative flours. Canned tomatoes, coconut milk, broths and spices enable quick cooking. Round it out with healthy fats, produce, herbs and flavor boosters like nutritional yeast.

Rotate stock:

Adopt the FIFO method - first in, first out. Keep newly purchased items behind current inventory. Use up existing items before opening new ones. This rotation system reduces food waste and ensures freshness.

Date items as you stock them. Establish a regular time to check expiration dates and clean out the pantry. Donate unopened items to food banks as they approach expiration.

Deep clean:

Do a deep clean every few months. Take everything out and wipe down shelves. Check for expired or unwanted items. Re-organize if needed to better fit your current diet and shopping habits. Do a thorough sweep for crumbs and spills that attract bugs. Restock with new groceries and enjoy the refreshed space!

An organized vegetarian pantry does require some upfront investment of time and supplies.

But the payoff is reduced stress, quicker cooking, and less food waste. Eating nourishing plant-based meals becomes simpler. Follow these principles for a high-functioning, efficient vegetarian pantry that makes your life easier.

FIFO

Reducing waste is an essential part of sustainable, eco-conscious vegetarian living. Adopting the FIFO (First In, First Out) method is an effective way to minimize discarded vegetarian foods. Here is a detailed overview of how to implement FIFO and enjoy its many benefits.

What is FIFO?

FIFO stands for First In, First Out. It is an inventory rotation system aimed at using up older stock first before newer stock. This ensures the oldest products get used before expiration dates cause spoilage.

How to Implement FIFO:

1. Arrange items with oldest in front: Place newly purchased items behind existing inventory. As you restock shelves, move older items to the front. Position them so they are most visible and convenient to grab.

2. Date items: Label all items with purchase dates as you stock them. Use stickers, tape or permanent marker for cans and boxes. For produce, use grease pencils directly on the

item. Dating helps clearly identify oldest versus newest.

3. Develop meal plans accordingly: Use your dated inventory to drive meal plans. Consult it as you menu plan and grocery shop. Incorporate soon-to-expire items into recipes first. Doing an occasional pantry cleanout will reveal which products need using soon.

4. Designate shelf life: Certain products have longer shelf lives than others. Know which vegetarian items last only weeks versus months or years. Prioritize cooking and freezing items closest to expiration. Eat fresh produce within prime ripeness and freeze any excess.

Benefits of FIFO:

1. Reduces food waste - By using up existing inventory first, less food gets pushed past prime freshness resulting in less waste. Planning meals around oldest stock ensures food gets eaten instead of discarded.

2. Saves money - There is less need to throw away spoiled or expired vegetarian products and rebuy. Making the most of what you already have reduces unnecessary grocery spending.

3. Achieves first in, first out flow - Having an effective stock rotation system means vegetarian ingredients get used at their peak. Oldest food gets eaten first while newest stock gets used later, preventing waste.

4. Maximizes shelf life - Adhering to FIFO ensures you enjoy the full shelf life of vegetarian items. Fruits, vegetables, breads, grains stay fresh longer when newest batches aren't left sitting behind old.

Tips for Success:

- Store vegetarian meats and cheeses in the coldest part of the fridge, not the door. Keep vulnerability to temperature in mind when organizing.

- Freeze soon-to-expire nuts, flours, or bread items to prolong life.

- Prep fresh produce soon after purchase - wash, chop, portion for easy grabbing.

- Avoid bulk purchases of perishable items you can't eat quickly enough.

- Do regular checks of dates and leftovers. Don't let items get forgotten.

- Get creative using up odds and ends - make soups, baked goods, veggie burgers.

Potential Challenges:

- Difficulty predicting usage and shelf life for new vegetarian products. You'll learn over time!

- Judging date labels - is it expiration, sell-by or best-by date? Know the difference.

- Household members not adhering to the FIFO system. Communicate the value!

- Resisting preparing food due to busy schedule. Prioritize FIFO-friendly meals.

The FIFO method does require a time investment upfront. But it quickly becomes habit and pays dividends through less waste. Not only is FIFO better for the planet, but your wallet too. An organized, date-conscious vegetarian pantry leads to reduced spoilage so food gets eaten, not discarded. Implementing FIFO simply takes dedication to using up what you have.

Building a Fresh Ingredient Routine

Incorporating an abundance of fresh produce takes vegetarian cooking to the next level. The right fruits, vegetables and herbs make plant-based meals colorful, flavorful and nutrient-dense. Follow these tips for shopping seasonal items and planning meals around nature's freshest bounty.

Benefits of Seasonal Produce:

Eating seasonally means enjoying fruits and vegetables at their peak freshness and ripeness. Produce harvested in season boasts superior flavor and nutrition compared to out-of-season options shipped long distances. Benefits of eating seasonal, local produce include:

- Maximum taste - Fruits and veggies straight from the source burst with natural flavors.

- Improved nutrition - Higher vitamin and antioxidant levels when produce is picked ripe.

- Supports local economy - Buying from nearby farms keeps money in the community.

- Reduced carbon footprint - Less resources used getting produce from farm to table.

- Cost savings - Seasonal items are plentiful, requiring less transportation and storage.

- Inspires creativity - Cooking with seasonal offerings pushes you out of recipe ruts.

Tips for Shopping Seasonally:

- Source from farmers markets - Ask farmers when crops will be at their best. Purchase small amounts frequently.

- Join a CSA (community supported agriculture) - Receive regular boxes of whatever is freshest.

- Read store signage - Many grocers now label produce with peak season and origin.

- Talk to store produce staff - Ask questions about seasonal arrivals and taste.

- Research online - Consult guides on harvesting timelines for your region's agriculture.

- Plan flexible menus - Don't get attached to specific items, be open to nature's offerings.

- Try new varieties - Sample heirloom and hybrids alongside classic choices.

- Embrace imperfection - Don't shy from slightly imperfect produce discounted to sell quickly.

Meal Planning Tips:

- Inventory your CSA box or market haul - Spark recipes from what you have on hand.

- Highlight what's ripe now - Then fill in with pantry items like grains, beans, oils.

- Swap ingredients freely - If you have chard swap it for kale in recipes.

- Preserve abundance quickly - Freeze, can or pickle seasonal surplus to enjoy year-round.

- Research preparation tips - Certain vegetables and varietals have specific cooking methods.

- Let nature guide you - Follow cravings and use more of what you enjoy most.

- Mix up flavors - Combine in-season ingredients in new ways.

- Stock up on staples - When you see seasonal finds like berries or ramps, buy extras to incorporate into various dishes.

Sample Seasonal Menus:

Spring - Asparagus tart with pea shoots, radish salad with chickpeas and lemon dressing, strawberry rhubarb crisp

Summer - Caprese salad with heirloom tomatoes, grilled corn and zucchini with chimichurri sauce, peach sorbet

Fall - Butternut squash soup, roasted Brussels sprouts with apples and pecans, pumpkin bread pudding

Winter - Sweet potato coconut curry, kale Caesar salad, blood orange scones

Eating according to season requires flexibility and creativity. But the rewards are well worth it - incredible flavors, nutrition, savings and sustainability. Follow these tips to stock up on garden goodness unique to each season and reap the benefits of fresh, local vegetarian ingredients.

Minimizing Waste

Adopting a vegetarian diet is a great sustainability choice. You can take it a step further by implementing strategies to minimize food waste. With some mindset shifts and smart practices, it's easy to repurpose ingredients and reduce what ends up in the landfill. Here are tips for meal planning, scraps usage, proper storage and more.

Meal Planning Strategies:

- Take weekly inventory of fridge, freezer and pantry items. Plan recipes to use up what you already have.

- Create a visual menu for the week. Schedule meals featuring perishable ingredients needing to be eaten soon.

- Double up on recipes that use versatile ingredients like beans, greens, grains and roasted veggies. Repurpose leftovers into new dishes later in the week.

- When groceries are delivered or bought, wash, chop, portion ingredients right away for easy grabbing all week.

- Freeze, preserve or pickle abundant seasonal produce to enjoy later. Bulk cook big batches of soups, chili and curries to freeze.

- Use parts of ingredients not typically consumed like beet greens and celery leaves in sautés, smoothies or stock.

Repurposing Scraps:

- Vegetable peelings, tops, stems and any unwanted parts can be saved to make broth.

Keep a bag in the freezer until you have enough to simmer into stock.

- Herb stems, garlic ends, onion nubs, wilted veggies and more also add flavor to stocks. Refrigerate scraps in an airtight container for 2-3 days max.

- Cheese rinds from harder cheeses impart delicious umami flavor when simmered into soups or sauces.

- Stale bread gets new life as bread crumbs, croutons, or used for stuffing, stratas or bread pudding.

- Overripe fruit is perfect for smoothies, chia puddings, or baking into muffins and cakes.

Banana peels can even be cooked into sweet treats.

Proper Storage Tips:

- Keep fridge below 40°F. Use a thermometer to monitor temperature and adjust as needed.

- Line produce drawers with paper towels to absorb excess moisture and prevent spoilage.

- Store greens, herbs and vegetables loosely wrapped or in breathable containers, not sealed in plastic bags.

- Transfer leftovers to airtight glass or stainless steel containers. Label with dates. Keep for 3-4 days max.

- Place new food items behind current inventory. Follow the FIFO (First In, First Out) system.

- Freeze food portions not eaten within a few days like sliced fruit, prepped veggies, soups, sauces.

- Wrap or cover foods well in the freezer. Use ice cube trays for small portions of sauces, herbs, veggie scraps.

With some forethought and basic best practices, it's simple to extend the life of perishable vegetarian ingredients. Repurposing odds and ends eliminates unnecessary waste. A vegetarian kitchen focused on sustainability utilizes the whole ingredient, composts inedibles, and masters smart storage. Eating

plant-based becomes even more earth-friendly.

Chapter Four

Breakfast

Vegan Shepherd's Pie

Ingredients:

For the bottom layer:

- ½ cup Cheddar soy cheese, shredded

- 14 oz pack vegetarian ground beef substitute

- 1 pinch ground black pepper

- 1 tsp Italian seasoning

- 1 large yellow onion, chopped

- ½ cup frozen peas

- 2 carrots, chopped

- 1 tbsp. vegetable oil

- 1 garlic clove, minced

- 1 tomato, chopped

- 3 celery stalks, chopped

  For the potato layer:

- ½ cup vegan mayonnaise

- 3 tbsp vegan cream cheese substitute

- 2 tsp salt

- ¼ cup olive oil

- ½ cup soy milk

- 5 russet potatoes, peeled and cubed

  Directions:

1. Place the potatoes in a pot. Add cold water and let it boil over medium heat until the potatoes are tender. Drain.

2. Combine the soy milk, salt, vegan mayonnaise, vegan cream

3. cheese and olive oil then add to the potatoes. Mash the potatoes until it is smooth. Set it aside.

4. Set the oven at 400 degrees. Coat the inside of a 2 quart baking dish with cooking spray. Place a large pan over medium heat then add the vegetable oil. Cook the tomato, onion, frozen peas, celery and carrots until tender. Season with the pepper, Italian seasoning and garlic.

5. Reduce the heat to low. Crumble the beef substitute and place in the pan. Cook for about 5 minutes until it is very hot.

6. Spread the meat substitute at the bottom of the dish. Spread the mashed potato on top.

Sprinkle the shredded soy cheese over the potatoes. Bake for 20 minutes until it is golden brown and the cheese is melted.

Black Bean and Tomato Soup

Ingredients:

- 2 carrots, chopped

- 1 large onion, chopped

- 1 15 oz cans black beans

- 1 pinch black pepper

- 14.5 oz crushed tomatoes

- 2 tbsp. chilli powder

- 15 oz can whole kernel corn

- 4 cups vegetable broth

- 1 tbsp ground cumin

- 4 garlic cloves, chopped

- 1 celery stalk, chopped

- 1 tbsp. olive oil

  Directions:

1. Pour the oil in a pan then place it over medium heat. Cook the carrots, garlic, celery and onion for 5 minutes.

2. Season it with cumin, black pepper and chilli powder. Cook it for a minute. Stir in 2 can of beans, corn and vegetable broth. Boil the mixture.

3. Process the remaining cans of bean until it is smooth. Add it to the soup mixture. Simmer

the mixture for 15 minutes until completely heated through.

Chinese-Style Fried Rice

Ingredients:

- 2 eggs Soy sauce
- 1/2 cup green peas
- 2 cups white rice
- 2 tablespoons vegetable oil
- 2/3 cup baby carrots Sesame oil
- 4 cups water

Directions:

1. In a large saucepan, bring water and uncooked rice to a boil.

2. Once the rice is almost cooked, reduce the heat, cover and simmer for about 20 minutes.

3. In another saucepan, boil the carrots for 5 minutes; add the peas.

4. Once the carrots are tender, drain the water, pour oil and cook for about 30 seconds.

5. Meanwhile, in a small bowl, beat the eggs and pour them in the saucepan.

6. Once you have scrambled the eggs, add soy sauce, peas, carrots and rice.

7. Add sesame oil and toss the rice before serving on a large dish.

Garlic Mashed Potatoes

Ingredients:

- 3 1/2 lbs. russet potatoes

- 16 fl. oz., half-and-half, around

- 2 cups 6 oz. Parmesan cheese grated

- 6 garlic cloves, crushed

- Kosher salt to taste

Directions:

1. Clean, peel and dice potatoes. Make sure that every chopped piece has virtually the same size. Transfer in a saucepan. Season with 2 tablespoons salt. Pour enough water to cover the potatoes. Set stove to medium-high heat and bring to a boil.

2. Reduce heat, but make sure the potatoes are still boiling. Check if potatoes are very tender by poking with a fork.

3. Combine garlic and half-and-half in a saucepan. Simmer over medium heat. Remove from stove and set aside.

4. Remove potato-filled pan from stove and drain water. Mash potatoes and stir in cream and garlic mixture. Add Parmesan cheese.

5. Continue stirring to combine every ingredient. Let it sit for 5 minutes for the mixture to thicken.

6. Serve a la carte or with a meat main dish.

Gourmet Style Sweet Potato

Ingredients:

- 5 sweet potatoes

- 2 eggs

- 1/2 cup butter, softened, divided

- 3/4 cup packed light brown sugar

- 1/2 cup white sugar

- 1 tsp. vanilla extract

- 1/2 cup pecans, chopped

- 3 tbsps. all-purpose flour

- 2 tbsps. heavy cream

- 1/2 tsp. ground cinnamon

- Salt

Directions:

1. Preheat oven (350 degrees Fahrenheit). Grease a 13x9-inch oven dish. Arrange sweet potatoes in another pan and bake for 35 minutes.

2. Once soft, take the pan out and let sweet potatoes cool. Peel then mash once it's cooled enough to handle.

3. Combine mashed sweet potatoes, vanilla extract, eggs, sugar, heavy cream, cinnamon, 1/4 cup butter, and desired amount of salt in a bow.

4. Mix then transfer into the greased baking dish.

5. Combine the remaining 1/4 cup butter, brown sugar, flour and pecans. Mix using hands to combine completely. Sprinkle on sweet potato mixture.

6. Bake for 30 minutes or until pecans are crispy and turned light brown.

Curried Brown Rice with Almonds

Ingredients:

- 1 pouch brown rice (pre-cooked)

- 1/2 cups red bell pepper

- 1/2 cup onion

- 1 teaspoon garlic

- 2 teaspoons yellow curry paste

- 1 tablespoon peanut oil

- 1 tablespoon fresh lime juice

- 1/4 teaspoon salt

- 1/4 cup cilantro leaves

- 1/4 cup almonds

Directions

1. In a wok, stir-fry the garlic and onions for about a minute then add the walnuts and bell peppers; cook for 2 minutes.

2. When the bell peppers have softened, add the rice and mix in the curry paste, salt, lime juice and cilantro leaves.

3. Toss the pre-cooked rice with the other ingredients and add peanut oil; keep warm.

4. Serve on a plate and top it with sliced almonds.

Red Lentil Soup

Ingredients:

- 1 cup dry lentils

- 1 pinch cayenne pepper

- 1 pinch fenugreek seeds

- 2 tbsp. tomato paste

- 1 pinch ground nutmeg

- 14 oz can coconut milk

- 1/3 cup cilantro, finely chopped

- 1 tsp curry powder

- 2 cups water

- 1 cup butter squash, peeled and cubed

- 1 tbsp fresh ginger root, minced

- 1 tbsp peanut oil

- 1 garlic clove, chopped

- Salt and pepper to taste

- 1 small onion, chopped

Directions:

1. Pour the oil in a large pot. Place it over medium heat. Add the garlic, onion, fenugreek and ginger. Cook and stir until combined.

2. Mix in the cilantro, lentils and squash. Add the tomato paste, water and coconut.

3. Stir the mixture thoroughly.

4. Season it with curry powder, nutmeg, salt, cayenne pepper and pepper.

5. Boil the mixture then reduce the heat for 30 minutes until the squash and lentils are tender.

Pumpkin and Spinach Salad with Mustard Vinaigrette

Ingredients:

- 1 butternut pumpkin

- 1/4 cup olive oil

- 300 grams baby spinach leaves

- 1 tablespoon mustard, wholegrain

- 2 tablespoons red wine vinegar

- 200 gram feta cheese

- 3 red onions

Directions:

1. Preheat your barbecue grill and set the temperature to a medium.

2. Cut the butternut pumpkin to several slices, brush with olive oil and season with pepper and salt.

3. Grill the pumpkin slices until they become tender and put on a plate.

4. On the same grill, add an onion and grill under it turns translucent then set aside.

5. In a large serving bowl, add the grilled pumpkin and onion, feta and spinach leaves.

6. Prepare the dressing by combining the vinegar, olive oil and mustard then pour the contents into a jar with a lid.

7. Toss the Butternut Pumpkin, Spinach Salad and serve with Mustard Vinaigrette Dressing.

8. Crumble some feta cheese for garnish.

Spinach and Berries Salad

Ingredients:

- Red wine vinaigrette

- 1/2 cup toasted almonds

- 1/4 red onion

- 2 bags baby spinach

- 1 package blue cheese

- 1 small bag of Strawberries Salt

- Pepper

   Directions:

1. In a small bowl, mix red onions, baby spinach, quartered fresh strawberries, crumbled blue cheese and toasted almond.

2. Drizzle the red wine vinegar and toss the vegetables to fully coat it.

3. Garnish with extra crumbled blue cheese and enjoy this light Summer Spinach and Berries Salad.

Spiced Soy Fried Rice

Ingredients:

- 1 bowl steamed rice

- 1 tsp coriander

- 7 cloves garlic

- 2 tsp oil

- 1 tsp soy sauce 1/2 tsp ginger

- 1 red chilli

- 1 egg Salt

- Pepper

  Directions

1. Heat a skillet and add 2 teaspoons of oil.

2. Add the egg and cook it for one minute but not after the yolk dries up.

3. Once the egg is done, set it aside and add the soy sauce, salt, red chili, pepper, garlic, and ginger.

4. Combine all ingredients including the cooked egg then add the steamed rice.

5. Toss well and serve with coriander leaves as garnish.

179

Deviled Eggs

Ingredients:

- 2 tablespoons sweet pickle relish

- 6 large eggs, hard-boiled

- 2 tablespoons classic salad dressing salt

- black pepper to taste

- 1 teaspoon yellow mustard

Directions:

1. Peel the shells off the cooled hard-boiled eggs and then slice into two, lengthwise.

2. Remove egg yolks from the whites and then transfer to a small mixing bowl.

3. Use a fork to mash the yolks into a fine crumble. Add 2 heaping tablespoonsful of yellow mustard, salad dressing or mayonnaise, sweet pickle relish. Season mixture with salt and black pepper to taste. Stir until creamy.

4. Spoon the mixture into a resealable sandwich bag. Seal the bag and then snip off one of its corners. Squeeze the mixture out of that corner, and into the egg white halves.

5. Keep in the refrigerator for about 1 to 2 hours, or until eggs are cold enough. Serve.

Sweet Deviled Eggs

Ingredients:

- 6 eggs

- 1 teaspoon hot mustard

- 1 tablespoon spicy brown mustard

- 2 tablespoons mayonnaise

- 1 teaspoon white sugar

- green olives, pimento-stuffed variety, halved

  salt

- pepper to taste

  Directions:

1. In a large saucepan, place the eggs and then cover with room temperature water to about an 1 inch above the eggs.

2. Cover saucepan and set heat to high, bringing the water to just a rolling boil. Remove pan from the heat. Just let the eggs stand in the hot water for about 15 minutes

3. Drain and then cool the eggs through cold running water. Once cold, peel eggs and then halve lengthwise.

4. Transfer egg yolks into a small or medium bowl and then mash using a fork. Stir in the spicy brown mustard, mayonnaise, hot mustard, salt, pepper, and sugar into the mashed yolks until thoroughly combined. Spoon the mixture into a resealable plastic bag with a one-quart capacity and then snip a corner off the bag.

5. Squeeze the yolk mixture into the egg halves, and then sprinkle paprika into each egg. Top with the halved olives. This makes 12 deviled egg halves.

Wasabi Cilantro Deviled Eggs

183

Ingredients:

- 1 dozen eggs

- 1/4 cup canola mayonnaise

- 4 teaspoons of wasabi paste

- 1/8 teaspoon black sesame seeds

- 2 tablespoons cilantro, chopped

- 4 teaspoons fresh ginger, grated

- 4 teaspoons of lime juice

- 1/4 sheet of nori, cut into small flakes

Directions:

1. Use a vegetable steamer to steam the eggs for 16 minutes. Allow to cool a bit and then peel. Slice the eggs in halves lengthwise, and then remove the yolks. Mash the yolks.

2. Stir lime juice, cilantro, mayonnaise, ginger, wasabi paste, and lime juice into yolks. Divide among egg whites before topoing with nori and black sesame seeds or ground chile.

Cream of Mushroom Soup

Ingredients:

- 8 oz. fresh mushrooms, chopped

- 2 qts. vegetable stock

- 2/3 cup flour

- 1 cup milk or half-and-half cream

- 6 tbsps. butter

  Directions:

1. Heat butter in a small pan or saucepan. Sauté mushrooms lightly.

2. Put flour and cook for 5 minutes while stirring constantly

3. Pour stock slowly. Stir until all ingredients are combined. Simmer for 10 minutes.

4. Pour cream and stir until blended. Serve.

Harvest Bread

Ingredients:

- 1 can (8 ounces) of crushed pineapple in juice

- 2 tablespoons oil

- 1/4 cup egg product, fat-free cholesterol-free or

- 1 egg

- 1 1/2 cups all-purpose flour

- 1/2 cup raisins

- 3/4 cup packed brown sugar

- 1 teaspoon baking powder

- 1/2 teaspoon salt

- 1/2 teaspoon baking soda

- 1/2 teaspoon cinnamon, ground

- 1 cup chopped walnuts

- 1 medium-sized carrot, shredded (about 1 cup)

- Cooking spray

Directions:

1. Heat oven to a temperature of 350°F.

2. Prepare loaf pan measuring 8 1/2x4 1/2x2 1/2 in inches by applying cooking spray. Drain crushed pineapples and then set aside.

3. Discard about 3 tablespoons of the juice from the crushed pineapple can. In a medium bowl, mix the remaining juice, egg product, oil and pineapple. Stir in the remaining ingredients

4. and then thoroughly blend. Spread this batter in the loaf pan.

5. Bake for 50 to 55 minutes. To check if bread is done, insert a toothpick in the center. It should come out clean. Allow to cool for about 10 minutes and then transfer bread from the pan to a wire rack. Allow to completely cool for around an hour before slicing. This makes 16 servings.

Gooey Caramel Bread

Ingredients:

- 2/3 cup of granulated sugar

- 4 cans of buttermilk biscuits, Refrigerated

- 2 teaspoons cinnamon

- 1 cup packed brown sugar

- 10 tablespoons of butter

Directions:

1. Heat oven to a temperature of 350°F. Prepare a 12-cup fluted tube pan by grease with shortening or applying cooking spray.

2. Place cinnamon and granulated sugar in a 1-gallon bag and then mix well. Separate the dough into biscuits and cut each in quarters using a pizza wheel (or a bread knife, if unavailable).

3. Shake the biscuit quarters in the bag to coat and then place in prepped pan. If there is any left in the sugar mixture, sprinkle them over the biscuits.

4. Place a 1-quart saucepan over medium-high heat and then bring brown sugar and butter to boiling point. Keep boiling for a

5. whole minute while constantly stirring. Pour sugar-butter melt over the biscuit quarters.

6. Bake biscuit quarters until golden brown, which usually takes 30 to 45 minutes. Cool for 5 minutes.

7. To serve, turn it upside down and then pull apart.

Raisin Rice Pilaf with Cheese and Cashews

Ingredients:

- 1 jar pimento peppers

- 1 and 1/2 cups long-grain white rice

- 1 cup chopped carrots

- 2 cups frozen green peas

- Ground black pepper

- 1 chopped onion

- 3/4 cup wild rice

- 1 cup golden raisins

- 3 cups vegetable broth 1 teaspoon salt

- 1 cup cashews

Directions:

1. In a large saucepan, add margarine, long-grain rice, raisins, carrots and onions.

2. Sauté the ingredients for 5 minutes then continue to simmer for 25 minutes to cook the long-grain rice.

3. Boil salted water in another saucepan and add the wild rice.

4. Cook it for 45 minutes and set aside to drain.

5. Wait until the basmati rice is done then add to the wild rice and cook it again for 45 minutes.

6. The Basmati and Wild Rice is now ready to be served with peas, cashew and pimentos on the side.

Sweet Potato Casserole

Ingredients:

- ½ cup pecans, chopped

- 1/3 cup all purpose flour

- ½ tsp vanilla extract

- 4 tbsp butter, softened

- 2 eggs, beaten

- 4 cups sweet potato, cubed

- 3 tbsp butter, softened

- ½ cup packed brown sugar

- ½ cup milk

- ½ tsp salt

- ½ cup white sugar

Directions:

1. Set the oven at 325 degrees. Place the sweet potatoes in a saucepan then add water. Cook at medium heat until it is tender. Drain then mash the sweet potato.

2. Combine the mashed sweet potato, eggs, salt, butter, white sugar, vanilla and milk. Whisk the mixture until smooth. Transfer the mixture in a baking dish.

3. Combine the flour and brown sugar in a bowl. Add the butter and stir the mixture until coarse. Add the pecans. Spread mixture on top of the sweet potato.

4. Bake it for 30 minutes until the top is golden brown.

Deep-Fried Mushrooms

Ingredients:

*   10 oz. fresh white mushrooms, cleaned by wiping

- 2 cups breadcrumbs,

- Panko if available

- 3/4 tsp. baking powder

- 1 cup flour

- 1 cup water

- 1/2 cup cornstarch Salt

  Directions:

1. Combine cornstarch, flour and baking powder. Add a dash of salt.

2. Pour water into the dry ingredients. Mix to form batter.

3. Dip mushrooms into the batter. Let excess mixture drip off.

4. Dredge mushrooms into breadcrumbs. Coat all sides evenly. Deep fry until golden.

5. Serve with preferred sauces like cocktail sauce.

Chapter Five

Lunch

Baked Ziti with Fire Roasted Tomatoes

Ingredients:

- 8 oz ziti, cooked and drained

- 1 medium zucchini, halved lengthwise

- 3/4 cup Daiya cheese, shredded

- 1 can diced fire roasted tomatoes, drained

- 1 cup sweet onion, chopped

- 2 cloves of garlic, finely chopped

- 1 15-oz can of tomato sauce

- 2 teaspoons fresh oregano leaves, chopped

- 1/4 teaspoon pepper

- 1/4 teaspoon salt cooking spray

  Directions:

1. Heat oven to a temperature of 375 degrees F. Grease a rectangular 2 quart glass baking dish with cooking spray.

2. In a 10-inch nonstick pan, cook onion, and garlic set over medium heat, constantly stirring until cooked. Add the zucchini pieces and then cook for 2 minutes.

3. Stir in the diced tomatoes, tomato sauce, salt, pepper and oregano. Heat to boiling point and then toss mixture with pasta.

4. Spread mixture in dish and then cover with foil. Bake for about 20 minutes and then sprinkle

with mozzarella. Remove cover and then bake for 5 more minutes until cheese melts.

Three-Cheeses Pasta

Ingredients:

- 1 16-oz package of ziti pasta, dry

- 6 ounces Daiya cheese, sliced

- 6 ounces vegan provolone cheese, sliced

- 1/2 cup hemp seed crumble cheese, grated

- 1 onion, chopped

- 2 jars spaghetti sauce

- 1 1/2 cups vegan sour cream

- 1/4 cup fresh basil, chopped

  Directions:

1. Pour water on large pot. Add some salt and bring to a boil and then add ziti. Cook for about 8 to 10 minutes or until pasta is al dente. Drain.

2. Brown beef in a large pan over medium heat. Add the onions and then sauté until softened. Drain off fat and then add the

3. spaghetti sauce. Lower heat to simmer for about 15 minutes.

4. Preheat oven to a temperature of 350 degrees F.

5. Lightly grease a 2 quart baking dish. Spoon in about half of the pasta and then top with a layer of provolone and mozzarella slices. Top with a layer of half the spaghetti sauce mixture and the sour cream, making sure to spread evenly.

6. Cover layer with what's left of the pasta, cheese slices, and sauce. Then, sprinkle a layer of Parmesan and basil.

7. Bake pasta in the oven until the cheese and sauce are bubbly, which should take around 30 minutes. This makes 8 servings.

Broccoli Pasta

Ingredients:

- 8 oz. thin spaghetti or linguine, cooked, rinsed and drained

- 1 tbsp. butter

- 2 1/2 lbs. fresh broccoli

- 1/3 cup olive oil

- 2 garlic cloves, minced

- 1 pinch cayenne pepper

- Hemp seed crumble cheese, grated

- Salt

- pepper

Directions:

1. Cut broccoli stems and florets into bite-size pieces.

2. Sauté oil, butter, garlic, broccoli, pepper and salt in a large pan over medium heat. Cook for 10 minutes while stirring frequently.

3. Plate pasta on a serving dish.

4. Top pasta with broccoli mixture.

5. Top with cheese.

Caramelized Butternut Squash

Ingredients:

- 2 butternut squash

- 6 tablespoons butter, unsalted

- 1/4 cup light brown sugar

- 1 and 1/2 teaspoons salt

- 1/2 teaspoon ground black pepper

Directions:

1. Preheat your oven to 400 degrees F.

2. Line a baking sheet with parchment paper or spray cooking oil.

3. Directly add pepper, salt, butter and sugar in the baking sheet, roast in the oven for 55 minutes.

4. While roasting the squash, occasionally turn them around for even browning.

5. Once done, season with pepper and salt; serve on a plate.

Squash Soup

Ingredients:

- 2 medium potatoes

- 1 container vegetable stock

- 1 onion

- 1 stalk celery

- 2 tablespoons butter

- 1 medium carrot

- 1 medium butternut squash

- Salt

- Pepper

Directions:

1. In a large pot, add the onions, potatoes, celery and squash; cook with butter for 5 minutes.

2. Pour vegetable stock over the vegetables and bring to a boil.

3. Once the mixture boils, reduce heat and simmer for 40 minutes.

4. Transfer the hot soup to a blender and blend until smooth.

5. Season with pepper and salt; serve immediately.

Broccoli Rice Casserole

Ingredients:

- 2 cups wild rice, uncooked

- 3 heads broccoli, cut into florets

- 1 cup panko bread crumbs

- 2 carrots, peeled, diced

- 1 lb button mushrooms, chopped finely

- ½ cup heavy cream

- 8 cups vegetable stock, low-sodium

- ½ cup coconut cream

- ¼ cup all-purpose flour

- 1 stick butter

- 1 onion, diced finely

- 2 stalks celery, diced finely

- 2 tablespoons parsley, minced

- 1 teaspoon salt

- 1 teaspoon pepper

Directions:

1. In a medium saucepan, pour 5 cups broth and add wild rice. Bring to a boil. Reduce heat and cook for 35 to 40 minutes or until rice is slightly tender and breaks open. Reserve for later.

2. Boil a pot of water and prepare ice water bath. Blanch broccoli in the boiling water until a bit crisp and bright green in color. Drain water and quickly plunge into the ice water bath to prevent overcooking. Remove from ice water, drain and set aside.

3. Melt 6 tablespoons butter in a large pot over medium heat. Sautee onions and mushrooms for 3 to 4 minutes or until liquid from mushrooms evaporate.

4. Stir in carrots and celery for 3 to 4 minutes or until vegetables are tender. Sprinkle flour over

the vegetable mixture and mix well to incorporate.

5. Cook for 3 more minutes or until mixture is thick. Stir in heavy cream and cook until thick. Season with salt and pepper. Adjust seasonings according to your taste.

6. Mix cooked rice and broccoli and transfer in a 2-quart baking dish. Scoop out vegetable mixture using a ladle and spread it evenly over the top until the whole surface is completely covered with vegetables.

7. Melt the remaining butter and pour in another bowl. Add bread crumbs. Toss until breadcrumbs are fully coated with butter. Sprinkle the breadcrumbs mixture on top of the casserole.

8. Cover casserole with foil and bake for 20 minutes. Remove foil and continue baking for 15 minutes or until top is brown. Remove from oven and garnish with parsley.

Pumpkin Casserole

Ingredients:

- 2 cups pumpkin puree

- ½ cup almond flour

- ½ cup butter

- 1 cup white sugar

- 1 cup cashew milk

- 1 teaspoon vanilla extract

- ¼ cup applesauce

- Ground cinnamon

Directions:

1. Preheat oven to a temperature of 350°F.

2. Mix pumpkin puree, sugar, evaporated milk, flour, vanilla, eggs, cinnamon, and melted butter together.

3. Spoon mixture into casserole dish and bake for 1 hour or until top is lightly brown.

Baked Potato and Sour Cream Soup

Ingredients:

- 2 potatoes, medium, baked and then cooled

- 2 tablespoons of vegan sour cream

- 2 cups vegetable stock

- 1/8 teaspoon pepper

- 1/4 cup vegan cheddar cheese, shredded

- 1 onion, green, sliced

Directions:

1. Peel the potatoes and then cut into half-inch cubes. Set aside half and then put the other half in a processor or blender. Add chicken broth and then cover blender. Process until consistency is smooth.

2. Pour processed potatoes into a saucepan. Then, stir in pepper, sour cream, and the potatoes you set aside. Cook over low heat settings until soup is heated through. Make sure not to let it boil.

3. Garnish soup with bacon bits, cheese, and onion. This makes 2 servings.

Creamy Vegan Macaroni and Cheese

Ingredients:

- 1 ½ raw elbow macaroni

- 5 tablespoons butter, divided

- 1 ½ cups almond milk

- ½ teaspoon salt

- 2 vegan cheese, cubed

- 3 tablespoons all-purpose flour

- ¼ teaspoon pepper

- 2 tablespoons bread crumbs, dry

- 1 cup cheddar cheese, shredded

Directions:

1. Melt butter in a saucepan over a medium heat. Once melted, throw in salt, pepper and flour.

Stir the ingredients until they develop a smooth consistency. While stirring, carefully add milk.

2. When all the milk has been added, leave on the flame to boil. Reduce the flame to low when the mixture becomes thick.

3. Cook the macaroni in a separate pan of boiling water according to the instructions on the pack. Drain the macaroni once done.

4. In a separate backing dish, transfer the cooked macaroni and pour the butter mix in with the macaroni and mix.

5. Bake the dish at 191C for about half an hour. This will result in the top of the mixture turning golden brown. This can now be served immediately.

Mushroom Stroganoff

Ingredients:

- 2 oz. dried dark mushrooms

- 1 lb. fresh, firm mushrooms

- 1 qt. hot water

- ½ medium-sized onion, minced

- 4 Tbs. butter

- Pinch of thyme

- 1 cup vegan sour cream

- 2 Tbs. brandy

- 1 lb. wide egg noodles

- 3 to 4 Tbs. butter, melted

- 3 tsp. poppy seeds

- salt

- fresh-ground black pepper

Directions:

1. Soak the dried mushrooms in a quart of hot water for several hours. Drain them, reserving the liquid. Wash the mushrooms thoroughly under running water, one by one, and trim off the hard stems.

2. Cut the mushrooms in wide strips. Strain the liquid through several layers of cheesecloth or through a paper coffee filter; there should be about 2 cups of it now. Transfer the liquid to a saucepan and simmer it until it is reduced by slightly more than half.

3. Meanwhile, wash, trim, and thickly slice the fresh mushrooms. Sauté the minced onions in the butter until they are transparent, then add the sliced fresh mushrooms and toss over high

215

heat until they have released their excess water and it is starting to evaporate. Season with a pinch of thyme and salt and pepper to taste. Add the soaked mushroom strips and reduce the heat to medium-low.

4. Gradually whisk the reduced mushroom liquid into the sour cream, and add this mixture to the mushrooms.

5. Simmer gently, stirring often, for 15 to 20 minutes, or until the sour cream sauce is slightly thickened and the mushrooms are tender.

6. Boil the noodles in a large amount of vigorously boiling salted water until they are just tender but not yet soft. Drain them

immediately and toss them with the melted
butter and poppy

7. seeds in a heated bowl.

8. Serve with the poppy seed noodles, and follow
it with a tart, crisp salad.

Mushroom Hazelnut Pilaf

Ingredients:

- 1/2 cup long-grain rice, uncooked

- 1/4 cup orzo pasta, uncooked

- 1/4 tsp. dried marjoram

- 2 cups vegetable stock

- 1/2 cup onion, chopped

- 1/2 cup hazelnuts, chopped, toasted

- 1/2 cup fresh mushrooms, sliced

217

- 1/4 cup celery, minced

- 1/4 cup butter

- 2 tbsps. fresh parsley, chopped

- Black pepper

Directions:

1. Melt butter in a pan over medium-low heat.

2. Sauté onion, mushrooms, rice, celery, and rice. Continue sautéing until rice is lightly brown.

3. Pour broth into the mixture and add hazelnuts, marjoram and parsley. Season with quarter teaspoon of freshly ground black pepper. Bring to a boil.

4. Reduce heat and cover. Simmer for 15 minutes.

5. Remove from stove and let sit for 10 minutes. Serve.

Stuffed Cabbage Rolls

Ingredients:

- 2½ lbs. fresh, ripe tomatoes

- 4 Tbs. olive oil

- 1 large onion, chopped

- 3 to 4 cloves garlic, minced

- 1½ tsp. paprika

- 1 large head green cabbage red wine

- salt pepper

Directions:

1. Place the whole head of cabbage in a large kettle and pour boiling water over it. In a few moments, the outer leaves will soften. Lift the

cabbage out and very gently peel off the soft leaves.

2. Repeat this procedure until all the leaves large enough to wrap around a spoonful of stuffing have been removed. If the cabbage leaves are not pliable enough to wrap and fold without tearing, douse them with boiling water again and leave them in it until they are soft.

3. Cut off the very stiff core ends and trim the largest leaves just a little. Place a rounded tablespoonful of stuffing near the thick end of a leaf. Fold the end over the stuffing, then fold over the sides, as if making an envelope.

4. When the sides are neatly tucked over, roll up the cabbage leaf as tightly as possible without squeezing out the stuffing.

5. Continue in this manner until all the stuffing is used. You should have enough for 12 to 15 cabbage rolls.

6. Blanch the tomatoes in boiling water and peel them. Purée them in a blender at low speed for a very short time—the resulting sauce should be thick and have bits of tomato in it.

7. Heat the olive oil in a large skillet and sauté the onions, garlic, and paprika in it until the garlic is golden. Add the tomato purée, a little red wine, and salt and pepper to taste. Simmer the sauce gently until it is thickened, at least ½ hour.

8. Lightly butter or oil a big, shallow (about 2 inches deep) baking dish. Put a few spoonfuls of the tomato sauce in the bottom.

9. Arrange the cabbage rolls in one neat layer in the dish. Pour the remaining tomato sauce over them.

10. Bake the cabbage rolls in a preheated 350 degree oven for about 40 minutes and serve piping hot.

Grilled Eggplant Salad

Ingredients:

- 1 eggplant
- 1 tomato, quartered
- 1 Tbsp. sherry vinegar
- ¾ tsp. smoked paprika
- 1 garlic clove
- 2 cups mixed baby lettuce

- 2 Tbsp. olive oil

- ¼ tsp. sea salt

- Olive oil cooking spray

  Directions:

1. First make the dressing by combining the tomato, garlic, vinegar, and smoked paprika in a food processor. Blend to combine, then add the olive oil and blend again to mix. Set aside.

2. Slice the eggplant into thin rounds and place in a colander. Salt the eggplant slices and toss to coat. Set aside for 10 minutes to dehydrate slightly.

3. Preheat the grill to medium flame.

4. Blot the eggplant slices with paper towels, then coat with olive oil cooking spray.

5. Grill the eggplant slices for 3 minutes per side, or until tender with grill marks.

6. Place the lettuce in a salad bowl and add half the dressing. Toss to coat then divide into two servings.

7. Divide the eggplant slices between the two servings, then drizzle the remaining vinaigrette on top. Serve right away.

Baked Stuffed Tomatoes

Ingredients:

- ¾ lb. green bell peppers (about 2 large)

- ¾ lb. zucchini

- ½ lb. small Japanese eggplants (about 3 eggplants)

- 1 small yellow onion

- ¼ cup olive oil

- 1½ tsp. salt, or more to taste

- 2 Tbs. chopped fresh cilantro (coriander leaves)

- 1 tsp. crushed dried red peppers

- dash of oregano

- 1½ Tbs. lemon juice

- black pepper to taste

- 8 ripe tomatoes

- ½ lb. Munster cheese, grated

- 2 Tbs. dry bread crumbs

- ¾ of the grated cheese.

Directions:

1. Roast the bell peppers under the broiler, turning them often, until they are blistered and charred. Hold them under cold running water and peel off the skins. Remove the stems, seeds, and ribs, and cut them in short, thin strips.

2. Trim and finely dice the zucchini and eggplants. Peel and chop the onion.

3. Heat the olive oil in a large skillet and sauté the chopped onions in it over very high heat, stirring constantly, just until they begin to color. Add the diced zucchini and eggplant and toss, still over high heat, for about 5 or 6 minutes. Add the salt, cilantro, red pepper, oregano, lemon juice, and black pepper. Stir well and turn off the heat.

4. Cut out a 2-inch circle from the top of each tomato and scoop out the pulp, leaving a ¼-inch shell. Chop the tomato pulp coarsely, add it to the vegetables in the skillet, and stir again over high heat just until the liquid is reduced to a thick paste.

5. Remove the vegetables from the heat and quickly stir in about

6. Spoon the mixture into the tomato shells. Toss the remaining

7. cheese with the bread crumbs and put a little mound of it on top of each tomato.

8. Bake the tomatoes in a preheated oven at 350 degrees for 15 to 20 minutes and serve immediately.

Chipotle Chowder

Ingredients:

- 2 red potatoes, diced

- ½ cup diced celery

- ½ cup diced carrot

- 2 Tbsp. chopped fresh parsley

- 2 garlic cloves, minced

- 3 cups vegetable broth, low sodium

- 2 ½ cups fresh sweet corn kernels

- 1 cup diced onion

- ¼ cup julienned red bell pepper

- 2 Tbsp. chopped chives

- 2 Tbsp. coconut oil

- 1 ½ Tbsp. minced chipotle pepper in adobo sauce

- 1 Tbsp. chopped fresh cilantro

- Freshly ground black pepper, to taste

Directions:

1. Place a soup pot over medium high flame and heat through. Once hot, add the oil and swirl well to coat.

2. Stir in the onion, carrot, celery, and garlic and sauté until the onion is translucent.

3. Add the diced potatoes and season with black pepper. Stir well for about 5 minutes, then add the corn kernels and chipotle. Stir well.

4. Pour in the coconut milk and vegetable broth. Bring to a boil, then reduce to a simmer and cover.

5. Simmer for 15 to 20 minutes, or until the potatoes are fork tender.

6. Allow the soup to cool slightly, then puree with an immersion blender or using a food processor. Then, stir in the chives and parsley. Reheat, if needed.

7. Ladle into soup bowls and top with bell pepper and cilantro. Best served right away.

Eggplant with Cheese and Nuts

Ingredients:

- 2½ lbs. firm eggplant

- 1 ⅓ cup walnut pieces

- 4 garlic cloves, sliced

- 2 red onions, sliced

- 3 cups peeled plum tomatoes

- ⅓ cup dry white wine

- ½ lb. Fontina cheese

- ¼ lb. mozzarella cheese

- ½ cup olive oil Salt

- Ground black pepper

  Directions:

1. Trim off the stem ends and slice the eggplants lengthwise, ½ inch thick. Salt the slices liberally on both sides and put them aside for about ½ hour to drain.

2. In a large skillet, sauté the garlic in the olive oil for several minutes, then remove and discard the garlic. Rinse the eggplant slices and press out the excess moisture between the palms of your hands. Brush the eggplant slices on both sides with the olive oil, and broil them for

several minutes on each side until they show dark spots.

3. When all the slices have been broiled, add to the remaining oil the sliced onions and stir over high heat until they are limp and beginning to brown. Cut the plum tomatoes in very thick slices and add them, with all their juice to the onions. Stir in the wine. Cook for several minutes over high heat, stirring often, and add about ½ teaspoon of salt and pepper to taste.

4. Pour the tomato sauce into a large, shallow casserole. Arrange the broiled eggplant slices over it in one even, overlapping layer. Sprinkle the slices with a little salt and pepper, then spread the walnut pieces evenly over the eggplant.

5. Cut the Fontina cheese in slices or strips and arrange it evenly over the walnuts. Grate the mozzarella and sprinkle it over the Fontina.

6. Bake the casserole in a preheated oven at 350 degrees for 20 to 30 minutes: It should be bubbling hot, and the cheeses should be melted and beginning to brown. Serve.

Grilled Mushroom Cheese Sandwich

Ingredients:

- 8 slices crusted bread

- 4 slices vegan cheese

- 1/2 lb. white mushrooms, sliced thinly

- 2 tbsps. butter

- 2 tbsps. Dijon mustard, optional

- 1 tbsp. fresh thyme

- Salt pepper

- butter and olive oil, for grilling

Directions:

1. Heat butter in a pan. Sauté mushrooms and thyme until golden in color. Season with salt and pepper.

2. Prepare four bread slices. Place a slice of cheese on each bread. Spoon 1/4 of the mixture for each slice.

3. Add mustard if preferred. Cover with the last bread slices.

4. Heat a bit of oil and butter in a grill pan.

5. Grill bread until grill marks appear or when cheese melts.

Spinach and Dill Rice

Ingredients:

- 1½ cups long-grain white rice

- ½ cup fresh-grated hemp seed crumble cheese

- 1 lb. fresh spinach

- 2 cloves garlic, minced

- 3 Tbs. olive oil

- 1 tsp. dried dill weed

- 2 tsp. white wine vinegar

- 4 cups water

- ½ cup finely crumbled feta cheese

- 2 tsp. salt

- fresh-ground black pepper to taste

Directions:

1. Wash and trim the spinach and mince it. Heat the olive oil in a small skillet and add the minced spinach and minced garlic to it. Season the spinach with ½ teaspoon of the salt, the dill weed, vinegar, and some black pepper.

2. Cook the mixture over medium heat for about 10 minutes, stirring often. All the excess liquid should have evaporated, leaving a thick purée.

3. Bring the water to a boil in a medium-large saucepan and stir in the remaining 1½ teaspoons salt. Add the rice and lower the heat to a simmer. Cover the pot and leave the rice to cook over very low heat for 25 minutes. The rice will absorb all the water.

4. Add the spinach mixture and toss lightly with two spoons until the rice and spinach are well blended. Cover once more and leave over low heat for another 3 to 4 minutes.

5. Toss together the 2 cheeses. Spoon the green rice onto a warmed platter, sprinkle it with the cheeses, and serve immediately.

Green Curry

Ingredients:

- 1 lb. potatoes

- 1 lb. green beans

- ¾ lb. zucchini

- 1 lb. spinach

- 5 Tbs. butter

- 1½ lbs. onions

- 10 medium-sized cloves garlic

- 2 tsp. ground turmeric

- 1 Tbs. ground coriander

- 1 Tbs. ground cumin

- ½ tsp. hot paprika

- ½ tsp. cayenne pepper

- ¼ tsp. cinnamon

- 1½ Tbs. peeled and grated fresh ginger

- 4 Tbs. chopped green chilis

- 2 Tbs. lemon juice

- ¾ cup water

- 1½ tsp. salt

- ½ tsp. black pepper

Directions:

1. Scrub or peel the potatoes, quarter them lengthwise, and slice thickly. Boil in salted water for 5 minutes only, drain, and set aside.

2. Trim the green beans and cut them in 1-inch pieces. Boil them in salted water for 5 minutes, drain, and set aside.

3. Slice the zucchini rather thickly, boil them in salted water for 3 to 4 minutes only, drain, and set aside.

4. Wash and coarsely chop the spinach and set it aside.

5. Melt the butter in a large pot. Halve and thickly slice the onions and crush or mince the garlic, and sauté them in the butter until the onions begin to color. Then add the turmeric,

239

coriander, cumin, hot paprika, cayenne, black pepper, cinnamon, and salt.

6. Stir this mixture over a medium flame for a few minutes, then add the prepared vegetables, the ginger, green chills, lemon juice, and water.

7. Stir all the vegetables and spices together thoroughly and simmer, stirring again frequently, until most of the water is gone and the vegetables are just tender.

Sweet Potato Bake

Ingredients:

- 2 cans of sweet potatoes in light syrup (29-oz ea), drained

- 1/2 cup of melted butter

- 1/2 cup of white sugar

- 1 teaspoon of vanilla extract

- 2 eggs, beaten

- 1/3 cup of milk

  For the topping:

- 1/2 cup of all-purpose flour

- 1 cup of brown sugar

- 1/3 cup melted butter

- 1 cup of pecan halves

  Directions

1. Preheat the oven to a temperature of 350 degrees Fahrenheit.

2. Mash the sweet potatoes. Then, stir in half a cup of melted butter, the sugar, vanilla, milk

and eggs. Keep stirring until consistency is smooth.

3. Pour mixture into a 9-in. x 13-in baking dish and then spread evenly. In another bowl, mix the first three topping ingredients thoroughly. Stir in pecans. Spread the topping over the sweet potatoes evenly.

4. Bake in the oven for around 25 minutes, until the top is golden and sweet potatoes are bubbly.

Chapter Six

Dinner

Garbanzo Bean Salad

Ingredients:

- 6 cups garbanzo beans, cooked and drained

- 1 cup olive oil

- ½ cup red wine vinegar

- 4 cloves garlic, minced

- 1 tsp. sugar

- 3 Tbs. liquid from cooking beans

- 1½ small red onions, peeled, quartered, sliced
  thinly salt to taste

- fresh-ground black pepper

  Directions:

1. Make a dressing from the oil, vinegar, garlic, sugar, salt, pepper, and bean liquid. While the beans are still quite warm,

2. combine them with the onions and pour the dressing over them.

3. Toss until all the beans are evenly coated, then put aside for several hours before serving.

4. Serve cool or at room temperature. To cook dried garbanzo beans: Soak the beans overnight in enough water to keep them covered, with a pinch of baking soda in it.

5. The next day, add more water if needed, salt it well, and bring it to a boil. Reduce the heat and

simmer the beans until they are tender, about 1 to 1½ hours.

Rotini Salad

Ingredients:

- 5 plum tomatoes, chopped coarsely
- 1 pack rotini wheel pasta
- 1 cup fresh mushrooms, sliced
- 1 cucumber, chopped
- 1 cup Italian dressing
- 1 cup sliced olives
- 1 pack tomato sauce
- 1 tbsp. fresh oregano leaves
- 1 tbsp. if fresh basil leaves, chopped

- 1 red onion, chopped

Directions:

1. Cook pasta according to package directions.

2. Drain and rinse with cold or tap water. Drain again.

3. Combine Italian dressing, tomato sauce, oregano and basil in a bowl. You can use fresh or dried oregano or basil leaves in different measurements indicated above.

4. Mix the ingredients.

5. Add the rest of the ingredients and toss.

6. Cover with foil or cling wrap and refrigerate for 2 hours until chilled. Can be refrigerated longer as long as not over 48 hour.

Lima Bean Salad

Ingredients:

- 2 cups large dry lima beans

- 1½ qts. water

- salt

- ⅓ cup olive oil

- ¼ cup white wine vinegar

- plenty of fresh-ground black pepper

Directions:

1. Put the beans in a large pot with the water and 1 teaspoon salt, bring to a boil, reduce the flame. Simmer the beans gently for about 1 hour, or until they are just tender. Drain them while they are still hot, reserving the liquid.

2. In a skillet, boil the bean liquid vigorously for a few minutes until it is substantially thickened. Measure out ⅔ cup of the thickened liquid into a bowl.

3. Add 1 tablespoon salt plus all of the other ingredients to the warm liquid and whisk until well blended and you have a smooth sauce.

4. Pour the sauce over the beans while they are still warm and mix them up gently with a wooden spoon, being careful not to mash them. Refrigerate for several hours.

5. Before serving, stir salad again so that all the beans are well coated with the dressing.

Greek-Style Pasta Salad

Ingredients:

- 1 box pasta salad mix

- 4 oz. feta cheese, crumbled

- 2 tomatoes, chopped

- 4 cups romaine lettuce, torn

- 1 cucumber, chopped coarsely

- 1 cup sliced olives

- 1/2 cup red onion, sliced thinly

- Oil or water as needed

Directions:

1. Prepare pasta as directed in the package. Combine oil, seasoning mix and water. Mix well.

2. Add pasta and the rest of the ingredients except cheese.

3. Toss to coat pasta and other ingredients with sauce. Top with crumbled feta cheese. Serve.

All Vegetables and Cheese Pasta

Ingredients:

- 2 cups tube pasta, uncooked

- 2 garlic cloves, minced

- 1/2 cup onion, chopped

- 1 cup Daiya cheese, shredded, divided

- 1/4 cup vegan ricotta cheese

- 2 cups yellow squash, chopped

- 2 cups tomatoes, chopped

- 1 cup zucchini, chopped

- 2 tbsps. fresh basil, chopped

- 1/8 tsp. red pepper, crushed

- ¼ cup applesauce

- 2 tsps. fresh oregano, chopped

- 1 tbsp. olive oil

- Butter, for greasing

Directions:

1. Preheat oven to 400 degrees F.

2. Cook pasta according to pack instructions without adding salt and oil. Drain and set aside.

3. Heat olive oil into a large pan over medium-high flame. Add onion and zucchini slices. Sauté for 5 minutes.

4. Add garlic and tomatoes then continue sautéing for 3 minutes. Remove from stove then add herbs and 1/2 cup mozzarella.

5. Season with salt and black pepper. Stir to combine ingredients. Mix applesauce and ricotta cheese in a small bowl. Season with salt.

6. Pour into the pasta mixture and stir.

7. Transfer all ingredients into an 8-inch square oven dish greased with cooking spray or other shortening.

8. Top with remaining Daiya cheese. Bake for 15 minutes until browned and bubbly.

Asparagus with Pine Nuts Pasta

Ingredients:

- 1 lb. asparagus, chopped diagonally

- 8 oz. pasta, uncooked

- 2 tbsps. lemon juice, freshly-squeezed

- 3 tbsps. pine nuts

- 1 tsp. garlic, minced

- 1/4 cup Parmigiano-Reggiano cheese, crumbled

- 2 tsps. extra virgin olive oil

- salt

- pepper

Directions

1. Preheat the oven to 400 degrees F.

2. Cook pasta as instructed in the package, but without adding oil and salt.

3. Put asparagus in the pasta on the last 3 minutes of cooking. Drain liquid.

4. Add minced garlic into the pasta-asparagus mixture and place back on stove. Toss well to combine.

5. Spread pine nuts in one layer on a jellyroll pan. Bake for 3 minutes until fragrant and golden in color. Stir occasionally. Transfer nuts to a small bowl.

6. Increase oven heat to 475 degrees Fahrenheit.

7. Arrange pancetta on the same baking pan. Bake for 6 minutes until crispy.

8. Mix olive oil and lemon juice in a small bowl. Season with salt and freshly ground black pepper then whisk.

9. Drizzle over pasta. Toss to coat all ingredients. Sprinkle with cheese and nuts. Serve.

Angel Hair Pasta with Garlic and Cheese

Ingredients:

- 8 oz. angel hair pasta

- 3 garlic cloves, sliced

- 1/4 cup olive oil

- 1/2 cup parmesan cheese, grated

- 2 tbsp. oregano

- 2 tbsp. rosemary

- 2 tbsp. thyme, chopped finely

- 1/8 tsp. chili pepper flakes Salt

- black pepper

Directions:

1. Boil water in a large pot.

2. Add a tablespoon of salt per 2 quarts water then do the other cooking procedures.

3. Heat oil over medium heat in a small saucepan. Sauté garlic herbs, pepper flakes, and parsley.

4. Add more pepper flakes if spicy pasta is preferred.

5. Sauté for a minute or until the ingredients are fragrant. Remove from stove.

6. Once the water is already boiling, add angel hair pasta and cook for 2 minutes or until al dente.

7. Drain pasta and rinse with cold water, just enough to stop pasta from further cooking. Make sure the pasta is still warm once transferred to a large bowl.

8. Top with garlic-herb mixture and toss to combine.

9. Top with parmesan cheese and several grinds of black pepper. Toss again. Serve.

Celery Root Salad

Ingredients:

- 1 lb. celery root

- 1½ qts. water

- ½ cup milk

- 2½ Tbs. mayonnaise

- 2 Tbs. lemon juice

- 1½ Tbs. white wine vinegar

- 2 tsp. Dijon mustard

- 1 Tbs. heavy cream salt

- pepper to taste

Directions:

1. Peel the celery root and cut it in julienne strips. Combine the water, milk, and lemon juice in a large saucepan and bring to a boil.

2. Add the celery root strips to the boiling liquid and leave them submerged until the liquid.

Quinoa Pilaf

Ingredients:

- 1 cup quinoa

- 1 onion

- 1 garlic clove

- 1 carrot

- 1 teaspoon olive oil

- 1 can vegetable broth

- 1/4 cup water

- 1/4 teaspoon salt

  Directions:

1. Prepare a non-stick large saucepan and lightly grease it with cooking spray.

2. Add the garlic, carrots, and onions and cook for 3 minutes.

3. Remove the first batch of vegetables and set aside.

4. Add quinoa, vegetable broth, salt and water in the carrot's pan and simmer for 15 minutes.

5. Fluff the rice and check if the carrots are already tender before transferring them on a plate. Serve while hot.

Cucumber and Olives Quinoa Salad

Ingredients:

- 1 cup quinoa

- 2 cups vegetable stock

- 1/4 cup green onion

- 1/2 cup red pepper

- 1/2 cup green pepper

- 3 ounces vegan feta cheese

- 1/2 cup cucumber

- 1/4 cup black olives

  For The Dressing

- 1 teaspoon garlic, minced

- 1/2 teaspoon oregano

- 1/4 cup lemon juice

- 2 tablespoons olive oil

- 1/2 teaspoon basil Pepper

Directions:

1. In a saucepan, boil the vegetable stock and add the quinoa.

2. Constantly stir the quinoa for 15 minutes before reducing the heat to a medium to low.

3. In a large bowl, place the quinoa when all the liquid is already absorbed and add the cheese and vegetables.

4. Prepare the dressing by whisking the olive oil, pepper, basil, lemon juice, garlic, oregano and salt.

5. Cover the quinoa with the dressing and plate the salad. Serve.

Spicy Quinoa and Garbanzo

Ingredients:

- 3/4 cup quinoa

- 11 can of garbanzo beans

- /2 cup toasted pine nuts

- 1 small onion

- 1/2 cup raisins

- 1/2 teaspoon black pepper

- 1 tablespoon olive oil

- 1/2 teaspoon cumin

- 1/2 teaspoon salt

- 1 1/2 cups chicken stock

- 1 1/2 teaspoons curry powder

- 1/4 teaspoon cinnamon

- 1 clove garlic

Directions:

1. In a saucepan, cook the garlic and onions in olive oil then stir in the salt, cumin, cinnamon, chicken stock, curry powder and pepper.

2. Add the quinoa to the mixture and boil for 20 minutes for it to cook.

3. After 20 minutes, check if the quinoa has absorbed the liquid; if it is nearly dried up; add the garbanzo beans, raisins and pine nuts.

4. Serve the Mediterranean Spicy Quinoa hot or at room temperature.

Lima Beans in Tomato Sauce

Ingredients:

- 1 lb. large dried lima beans

- 3 peeled tomatoes, coarsely chopped

- ½ to 1 tsp. rosemary, crushed

- 3 Tbs. olive oil

- 5 cloves garlic, minced

- 3 Tbs. onion, minced

- 1 tsp. salt

- ¼ cup lemon juice

- 2 cups thick tomato purée

- 1 tsp. sugar

- fresh-ground black pepper, to taste

Directions:

1. Put the lima beans in a large pot with about 2 quarts of water and some salt. Bring the water to a boil, then reduce the heat, and simmer the beans until they are tender, but don't let them get mushy. Drain them, and save the broth to use in a soup— it's delicious.

2. Heat the olive oil in a very large skillet and sauté the garlic and rosemary in it for a few minutes. Add the tomato purée, chopped tomatoes, red wine, salt, lemon juice, sugar, and a generous amount of black pepper. Simmer the sauce, stirring often, for about 15 minutes.

3. Add the drained lima beans and continue simmering, stirring now and then with a wooden spoon, for another 5 to 10 minutes. The sauce should be quite thick.

4. If you want to serve the lima beans hot, stir in the minced onions shortly before serving. If you want to serve them cold, as a salad, allow them to cool before stirring in the minced onions and chill them for a few hours or overnight—the flavor improves.

Chapter Seven

Snacks

Hearts of Artichoke and Palm Crepes

Ingredients:

- 12 crêpes

- 2 cups cooked artichoke hearts, sliced

- 1½ cups hearts of palm, sliced

- 2½ tsp. sugar

- 5 Tbs. butter

- 2 Tbs. lemon juice

- 1 egg, beaten

- salt

- Hollandaise Sauce

Directions:

1. Cut the artichokes in half, scoop out the chokes, and slice them thinly. Slice the hearts of palm about ¼ inch thick, cutting them in half lengthwise first if they are very thick.

2. Melt the butter in a large skillet and heat the vegetables in it, stirring constantly, for about 10 minutes. Add the lemon juice and sugar, and some salt if it is needed, and stir again.

3. Remove the vegetables from the heat and quickly stir in the beaten egg. The heat of the vegetables will cook it slightly. Continue stirring for a minute or two.

4. Divide the mixture among the crepes, putting about 2 rounded tablespoonful down the center of each one.

5. Roll the crepes up over the filling and sauté them in butter briefly on both sides before serving—just long enough so that they are hot through and lightly browned. Serve them with warm Hollandaise Sauce and a fresh fruit salad.

Applesauce Crepe

Ingredients:

- 12 Basic Crepes
- 2 cups applesauce butter for the pan
- ¼ cup sugar

Directions:

1. Spread 1½ tablespoons of the applesauce over half a crepe and fold the other side over it.

2. Spread another tablespoon of applesauce over half the surface of the folded crepe, and fold it in half once more. The crepe will be folded in a triangle, with a layer of applesauce between each layer of crepe.

3. Fill all the crepes in this manner. Shortly before serving, sauté the crepes in butter for a few minutes on each side, until they are golden brown and hot through.

4. Put two of the folded crepes on each dessert plate and sprinkle each serving with about 2 teaspoons sugar. Serve.

Baked Apples

Ingredients:

- 6 large baking apples, cored
- ⅔ cup flour
- ½ cup butter
- 1 lemon rind, grated
- ⅔ cup brown sugar
- heavy cream, vegan safe, chilled
- ½ cup raisins, chopped
- ½ tsp. cinnamon
- ¼ tsp. nutmeg
- ¼ cup curaçao
- ¼ cup water

Directions:

1. Cut out a generous round cavity in each apple but not breaking through the bottom.

271

2. Mix together the flour and brown sugar and cut in the butter with a pastry blender or work it in with your fingers. Add the

3. lemon rind, cinnamon, nutmeg, and raisins and mix thoroughly. Stuff the apples with this mixture.

4. Arrange the apples in a medium-sized, shallow casserole.

5. Combine the brandy, curaçao, and water, and pour the liquid over the apples.

6. Bake the apples in a preheated oven at 400 degrees for 40 to 45 minutes, basting them with the liquid every 6 or 7 minutes.

7. The filling will puff up and form hard little caps on top where the sugar caramelizes. When you take the apples out of the oven, let them cool

for about 15 minutes, then cut the stiff, dark-brown sugar crusts off of the filling, leaving just the soft, tender part.

8. Spoon any remaining liquid over the warm apples. Serve them either warm or cool, with heavy cream.

Peaches and Cream

Ingredients:

- 4 medium-sized peaches

- ½ large lemon juice

- 3 medium-sized bananas

- ⅛ tsp. cinnamon

- 1 cup heavy cream

- ⅓ cup confectioners' sugar

- ⅓ cup slivered almonds, blanched

- 2 tsp. powdered sweet chocolate

Directions:

1. Peel the peaches as thinly as possible and slice them in thin wedges. Peel and slice the bananas.

2. Toss the fruit gently in a bowl with the lemon juice, then add cinnamon. Toss again until evenly coated, then refrigerate for ½ to ¾ hours.

3. Whip the cream with the confectioners' sugar until it holds fairly stiff peaks.

4. Put the fruit and brandy mixture in an attractive, shallow serving bowl and sprinkle it with the slivered almonds.

5. Spoon the whipped cream over the fruit in swirls and peaks. Through a fine sieve, sprinkle on the powdered chocolate. Serve.

Pineapple and Mandarin Oranges Cake

Ingredients:

- 1 can crushed pineapple, unsweetened

- 1 can of mandarin oranges

- 1 package instant vanilla pudding mix

- 1 package frozen whipped topping

- 1 package yellow cake mix

Directions:

1. Preheat your oven to 350 degrees F.

2. Prepare two round pans; line them with parchment paper and set aside.

3. In a medium-sized bowl, add one package instant vanilla pudding mix with pineapples, eggs and water; mix until smooth.

4. Add all the oranges from the can; fold in the pudding mix batter.

5. Divide the batter and pour into the lined round pans; bake in the oven for 30 minutes.

6. Once the cakes are done, remove them from the pans and transfer to wire racks to cool down.

7. Spread the whipped toppings on over the cakes and refrigerate for 30 minutes.

8. Once the frosting is chilled, serve and slice the Mandarin Oranges and Pineapple Cake.

Sponge Cake

Ingredients:

- 6 eggs, separated

- 1½ tsp. baking powder

- 1 cup sugar

- ¼ cup boiling water

- 1 Tbs. lemon juice

- ½ tsp. vanilla extract

- 1½ cups flour

- pinch of salt

- 4 Tbs. butter, melted and cooled

  Directions:

1. Beat the egg yolks until they are creamy and light, then gradually add the sugar a bit at a time, while you continue beating.

2. Beat the yolks and sugar together until the mixture is pale colored and fluffy—another 10 minutes or so. Gradually add the boiling water, lemon juice, and vanilla and beat another few minutes.

3. Sift together the flour and baking powder and fold it into the egg yolk mixture. Beat the egg whites with a pinch of salt until they hold firm peaks and fold them gently into the batter, using as few strokes as necessary.

4. Pour the melted, cooled butter over the batter, leaving out the milky sediment at the bottom of the pan. Again, using as few strokes as

necessary, in order not to deflate the egg whites, scoop in the butter.

5. Spoon the batter into a buttered and floured 9- or 10-inch springform cake pan. Smooth the batter lightly in the pan.

6. Bake in a preheated oven at 325 degrees for 40 to 45 minutes if you're making 1 large cake, slightly less time if you're making 2 layers. The cake is done when it is golden on top and shrinking away from the sides and when a toothpick inserted in the cake comes out clean.

7. Let the cake cool in the pan for a few minutes, then transfer to a rack until it is completely cool.

8. Sponge cake, as its name indicates, is ideally suited for all those splendid tortes and desserts

in which a quantity of rum or brandy is meant to be soaked up by the cake layers.

Lemon Torte

Ingredients:

- 1 ⅔ cups ground almonds, unblanched
- 2 cups confectioners' sugar
- 2 Tbs. cornstarch
- 1¼ cups egg whites
- ¼ tsp. almond extract
- Lemon Filling
- blanched almond halves, for garnish

Directions:

1. Beat the egg whites with 1 cup of the confectioners' sugar until they hold soft peaks. Sift together the second cup of sugar and the cornstarch, add it to the egg whites along with the almond extract, and continue beating until the egg whites are stiff.

2. Fold in the ground almonds. Butter and flour two 10-inch cake pans and divide the beaten egg white mixture between them,

3. spreading it as flat and smooth as possible. Bake the layers in a preheated oven at 275 degrees for 1½ hours. They should be pale gold in color and shrinking away from the sides of the pan.

4. Allow the layers to cool slightly in the pans, then carefully remove them and let them finish cooling on racks.

5. Spread a little more than half the lemon filling on one layer and place the second layer on top of it. Spread the remaining filling over the top and sides of the top layer, leaving the sides of the bottom layer exposed.

6. Decorate the torte very simply with a few blanched almond halves or just swirl the lemon topping evenly with a butter knife and leave it plain. Chill the torte for at least an hour.

Pumpkin Muffins

Ingredients:

- 2 eggs, large

- 1 cup all-purpose flour

- 1 cup canned pumpkin

- 1 cup pastry flour, whole-grain

- 3/4 cup buttermilk, low-fat

- 3/4 cup packed dark brown sugar

- 1/4 cup pumpkin seeds, raw and unsalted

- 1/4 cup canola oil

- 3 tbsps. unsulphered molasses

- 1 tsp. vanilla extract

- 1 tsp. ground cinnamon

- 1 tsp. baking soda

- 1/2 tsp. ground ginger

- 1/2 tsp. salt

- 1/4 tsp. ground cloves

- 1/8 tsp. ground nutmeg

- Cooking spray

Directions:

1. Preheat oven to 400 degrees F.

2. Grease a 12-cup muffin pan with shortening or cooking spray.

3. Combine all the flour ingredients, salt, cloves, nutmeg, ginger, salt, cinnamon and baking soda in a bowl. Whisk to combine well. Set aside.

4. Combine sugar, oil, one egg and molasses in a large mixing bowl. Whisk until everything is completely combined.

5. Add another egg to the sugar-molasses mixture. Whisk. Stir vanilla and canned pumpkin.

6. Add flour mixture in two batches. Continue whisking until completely mixed. Pour batter on muffin cups. Top muffin batter with pumpkin seeds.

7. Nudge the pan on the counter several times to clear air bubbles inside the cups.

8. Bake for 20 minutes. Pierce the center part of muffin with a cake tester. Muffins are cooked once stick comes out clean. Continue baking otherwise.

9. Place muffin pan on a wire rack for 15 minutes to cool. Loosen muffins from cups by running a knife on its edges.

10. Remove from mold and let it cool completely on the wire rack.

Pecan Banana Muffins

Ingredients:

- 2 eggs

- 4 bananas, overripe

- 2 cups all-purpose flour

- 1 cup brown sugar

- 1/2 cup pecans, chopped

- 3/4 cup butter, unsalted, melted and cooled

- 1 tsp. vanilla extract

- 1/2 tsp. salt

- 1 1/2 tsps. baking soda

Directions

1. Preheat oven to 375 degrees F.

2. Grease muffin cups on two muffin pans.

3. Combine flour, salt and baking soda in a large bowl. Mix well by using a pastry blender or fork. Set aside.

4. Mash two bananas using a fork in a bowl. Mix the remaining two bananas and sugar using a handheld or counter top electric mixer for 3 minutes.

5. Add vanilla, eggs and melted butter to the banana-sugar mixture. Beat well. Scrape sides of the bowl to place the ingredients near to the mixing blade.

6. Add dry ingredients then blend. Pour mashed bananas and pecans to the mixture. Fold using a rubber spatula.

7. Scoop the batter into muffin cups. Fill each cup halfway. Nudge the pan on the countertop to eliminate air bubbles.

8. Cook for 20 minutes or until cake tester or a barbecue stick comes out clean when the muffin is pierced.

9. Take the pan out to cool and serve at room temperature or warm.

Corn Muffins

Ingredients:

- 3 cups all-purpose flour

- 2 eggs, extra large

- 1/2 lb. butter, unsalted, melted

- 1 cup cornmeal

- 1 1/2 cups almond milk

- 2 tbsps. baking powder 1 cup sugar

- 1 1/2 tsps. salt

Directions:

1. Preheat oven to 350 degrees F.

2. Line 12 muffin cups using paper cups.

3. Combine cornmeal, sugar, salt, flour and baking powder in a mixer. Use a paddle attachment to mix ingredients together.

4. Mix melted butter, eggs and milk in another bowl. Set the mixer to low speed then pour the milk mixture to the dry ingredients. Continue mixing until blended.

5. Fill muffin paper cups with butter to the rim. Bake for 30 minutes or until cake tester comes out clean and the tops are brown and crisp.

6. Take out of the oven and let it sit to cool. Unmold from the pan and serve.

Cheesy Tomato Muffins

Ingredients:

- 8 flaky biscuits

- 1 container grape tomatoes, chopped

- 1 cup vegan-safe cheese, grated

- 6 oz. vegan cream cheese, softened

- 1/2 cup onion, diced

- 1 tsp. mayonnaise

- 1/2 tsp. dried rosemary Salt

- Pepper

  Directions:

1. Preheat oven to 350 degrees F.

2. Use aluminum foil to line a rimmed baking sheet.

3. Grease with cooking spray or other shortening. You can also use a non-stick aluminum foil.

4. Press biscuits into a pan. They are enough to form eight cups.

5. Combine mayonnaise, rosemary, cream cheese, and a dash of salt and pepper in a bowl. Add onions and tomatoes. Mix together.

6. Scoop equal amounts of mixture into the biscuits. Top with cheese.

7. Wrap each biscuit loosely with foil, ensuring the foil won't touch the cheese.

8. Bake for 5 minutes until bacon is cooked and sizzling.

9. Remove from oven then let it sit to cool for 5 minutes before serving.

Apple Pudding

Ingredients:

- 3 large tart green apples

- ¼ tsp. ground cloves

- 3 Tbs. sugar

- 4 Tbs. butter

- ½ tsp. cinnamon

- 1 tsp. grated lemon rind

- 3 eggs

- 3 Tbs. sugar

- ½ cup flour

- 1½ cups milk

- ½ tsp. vanilla extract dash of nutmeg

- ¼ to ½ cup confectioners' sugar

Directions:

1. Quarter, peel, and core the apples and cut the quarters in thin slices. In a shallow, fireproof casserole, sauté the apple slices in butter for several minutes.

2. Add the sugar, cinnamon, cloves, and lemon rind and continue to cook the apples, stirring often, for another 5 minutes, or until the apples are just tender.

3. Beat together the eggs, flour, milk, sugar, vanilla, and nutmeg, or blend them in a

blender. Pour the batter over the apples and bake the pudding for 25 to 30 minutes in a preheated oven at 400 degrees, or until it is puffed and golden brown on top.

4. Sift confectioners' sugar over the top of the pudding and serve it warm with coffee or milk.

Sweet Pastry Crust

Ingredients:

- 1 ⅓ cups flour

- 1 Tbs. sugar

- ¼ tsp. salt

- ½ cup butter

- scant ⅓ cup ice water

Directions:

1. Sift together the flour, sugar, and salt in a mixing bowl. Slice the cold butter rapidly and drop the slices into the flour mixture.

2. With a pastry blender or two sharp knives, cut in the butter until the mixture resembles coarse corn meal.

3. Sprinkle the ice water over the flour-butter mixture and stir it in quickly with a fork, until the dough gathers together.

4. Form the dough into a ball, wrap it in waxed paper or foil, and chill it for about 2 hours.

Pumpkin Bread Pudding

Ingredients:

- 1 teaspoon ground cinnamon

- 3 cups almond milk

- 1 can of pumpkin

- 6 cups bread cubes

- ½ cup pecans, chopped

- 16 pecan halves

- ½ currants

- 3 eggs

- 1 teaspoon vanilla

- ½ teaspoon nutmeg, ground

- 1 cup brown sugar

Directions:

1. In a large bowl, combine all of the ingredients but leave out the pecans, currants and bread cubes. They will be added at a

2. separate time. Mix all of the ingredients together until they are well-combined. This is when currants, pecans and bread cubes will come in. Continue mixing until there is uniform thickness.

3. Pre-heat oven to a temperature of 350 degrees F.

4. Pour the contents of the bowl into a springform pan. Be sure that the inner sides of the pan have been greased to prevent sticking. Place the pan in an oven that has been pre-heated to 177C.

5. Bake the mixture for about an hour. A knife or toothpick can also be inserted to the pudding to see if it is already done. The pudding will be ready to eat when the toothpick comes out

clean from the pan. Can be served both warm

and refrigerated.

Conclusion

This vegetarian cookbook represents a project crafted with love and intention—to guide and inspire you as you embrace the plant-based lifestyle. Whether you're just dipping your toes into meatless meals or have already immersed yourself in vegetarian eating, it is my hope that this book has provided a sturdy foundation to equip your journey.

As you've cooked your way through these pages, a world of possibility has opened up, revealing the immense variety and versatility within vegetarian cuisine. From cozy breakfasts to satisfy any time of day, to hearty dinners chock full of flavor and nutrition, to tempting snacks and sweet treats, each thoughtfully designed recipe highlights the vibrant taste and wholesome goodness of plant-based ingredients. Incorporating these dishes into your routine marks a meaningful step toward enhancing health, treading lighter on the planet, and promoting compassion for animals.

Yet this cookbook aims to offer much more than a collection of recipes. It seeks to empower you with indispensable cooking techniques, practical tips, and the confidence to get creative in the kitchen. You've learned how to maximize flavors, retain nutrients, and build balanced, crave-worthy meals tailored to your tastes. You've gained insight into selecting quality ingredients, planning weekly menus, and harnessing the benefits of seasonal produce. Armed with this knowledge, you have all the tools to continue your culinary explorations and make each recipe your own.

Adopting vegetarianism transcends just the food on our plates—it embodies a lifestyle fueled by compassion, mindfulness, and reverence for nature's gifts. With each plant-powered meal you prepare, you create positive ripples, enhancing your own health and the wellbeing of the planet. Every ingredient, technique, and final dish carries opportunity to inspire others and contribute to a sustainable future.

Remember, this book marks merely the beginning of your journey with vegetarian cuisine, not the end. Continue seeking out new flavors, ingredients, and cooking methods to try. Find joy in sharing meals with loved ones and let your passion for plant-based foods motivate those around you.

As you grow and progress on this rewarding path, may this cookbook serve as a trusted companion, spurring you on with inspiration when needed. Please, take these recipes and make them your own—tweak them, adapt them, modify them to satisfy your unique tastes and needs. Embrace the freedom and creativity vegetarian cooking allows. Most importantly, savor the process of nourishing yourself and others with food made from an abiding place

of care.

Printed in Great Britain
by Amazon

32279655R00169